# THE SIX-WEEK
# bikini
# COUNTDOWN

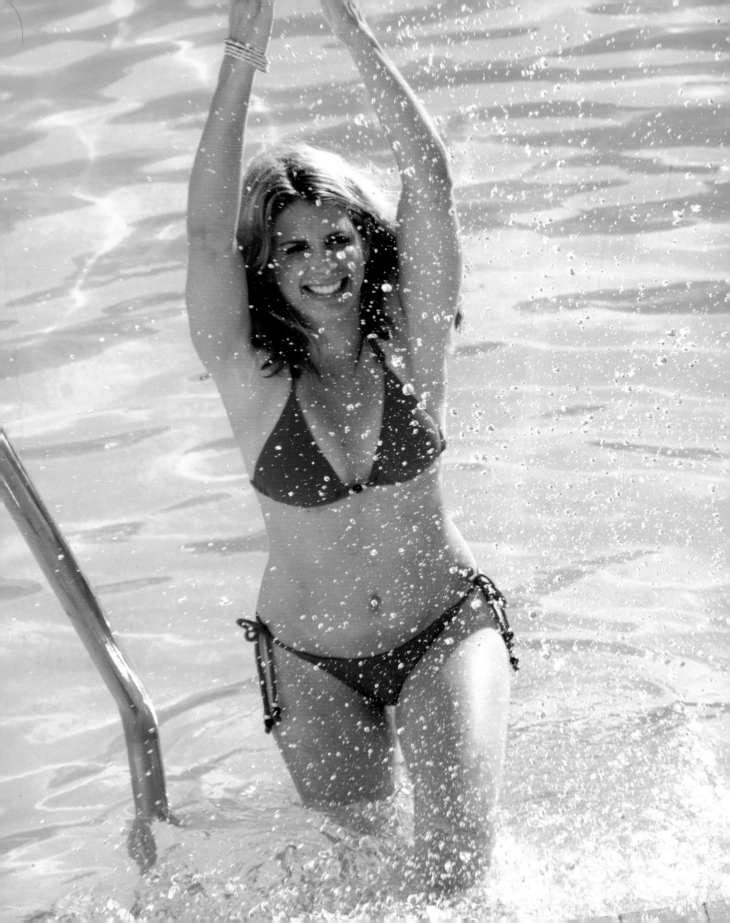

# THE SIX-WEEK

# bikini

# COUNTDOWN

Tone Your Butt, Abs, and Thighs Fast
Combining Pilates with Select Strength and
Cardio Interval Training Workouts

## karon karter

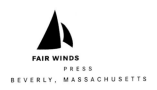

FAIR WINDS
PRESS
BEVERLY, MASSACHUSETTS

This book is dedicated to my father

(I'm sure you get the irony, Dad).

Text © 2008 Karon Karter

First published in the USA in 2008 by
Fair Winds Press, a member of
Quayside Publishing Group
100 Cummings Center
Suite 406-L
Beverly, Massachusetts 01915-6101
www.fairwindspress.com

12 11 10 09 08      3 4 5

ISBN-13: 978-1-59233-295-3
ISBN-10: 1-59233-295-1

Library of Congress Cataloging-in-Publication Data available

Cover design by Laura McFadden
Book design by doublemranch.com
Photography by Jack Deutsch

Printed and bound in Singapore

The information in this book is for educational purposes only.
It is not intended to replace the advice of a physician or medical practitioner. Please see your health care
provider before beginning any new health program.

# contents

# acknowledgments

With every ounce of gratitude in my bikini body, I would like to thank Will Kiester, my publisher. Of all the fitness experience I gathered throughout my lifetime, the too-many-hours-to-count teaching, the twenty-hour weekend workshops, and the six-day-a-week workouts (even when I didn't want to)—it was all for this book. As with my own body, this book has gone through some changes (the title changed several times) but I never gave up on my vision of blending Pilates with traditional fitness because I strongly believe you need it all to feel great and keep your body healthy. Will trusted me to write my vision—he's the best!

Behind every great man is a team of women! My gratefulness extends to the entire editorial team: my development editors, Tere Stouffer (she pulled a few all-nighters to edit my book and write her own—she's amazing) and Cara Connors (always sweet and patient); Tiffany Hill (editorial assistant); and Karen Levy (copyeditor). I'm indebted to John Gettings for making sure my book graces the bookshelves. And, of course, there wouldn't be a book without Ken Fund (the big boss). Three books later and it's wonderful being part of your team. Thank you for everything.

On the creative side, every girl needs a Rosalind Wanke, the best art director in the industry. I'm truly a lucky girl to work with her and one of the most dedicated photographers, Jack Deutsch. Together, we sweated it out in Miami in August during our four-day photo shoot. Despite the oppressive heat, Sheika Daley (makeup artist from the Ford Model Agency) did her best to make me look fresh though I was a dripping mess and Jack's oh-so adorable photographer's assistant, Federico Velez, went out of his way to make sure I was comfortable even though the sun was bearing down on me. Thank you all!

Those beautiful clothes came from my favorite line of clothing Lululemon Athletica–thank you so much Joanna Waller! And those sexy swimsuits came from Everything But Water–thank you Brenda Hernandez and Maryam Sakhai for your honest opinions. Of course, I wouldn't have a book without my students because they have done and loved every exercise in this book. Thank you to my personal trainer (trainers need trainers, too), Naz Habibi. She played a valuable role in helping me with the strength moves, which is her specialty. And finally, my agent Marilyn Allen, you're wonderful for being so patient and kind.

Lastly, on the most important topic, I am blessed to have a wonderful family and friends. My mother blends both grace and dignity. I love you Donna for doing my bikini program *and* proving that it works. You look oh-so smoking hot! Oh, and then there is my aunt Pat, who at age 62, still looks beautiful in her bikini–you go girl!

# introduction

Welcome to Your Bikini Crash Course. It's time to unveil the sexy vixen hidden underneath your baggy sweats and show off your bikini body. Don't worry if you have a little cellulite (what woman doesn't?) or you're carrying a bit of a belly around the middle. With The Six-Week Bikini Countdown, you won't be saddled by saddlebags or burdened by your underbutt any longer. Instead, your abs, legs, and butt will be better than ever, and you can stroll the beach with confidence. I'm not just talking about any old confidence, but a certain "I'm hot" type of confidence that will turn up the heat on the beach and turn you into a beach babe. The Six-Week Bikini Countdown is your crash course to your sexiest bikini body, and that's a promise.

Why six weeks? Because you can get lean all over in that amount of time. The truth is, I do it every bikini season. As a fitness writer and Pilates instructor, exercising and eating healthily are part of my routine and lifestyle, but sometimes I just need a break, usually around the holidays. After a couple of weeks of stuffing myself, I'm ready to work it all off. I don't beat my beat myself up about gaining a few pounds, instead I get bikini motivated! But I'm not going to sugarcoat it: the only way to get into shape is to burn calories and build muscle to fight fat. Diets don't work, but hard work does. Muscles are beautiful. Strong bodies, working out and eating healthily, are just plain sexy.

You'll work hard in these six weeks, substituting some of my routines for your regular workouts to burn more calories and sculpt more lean muscle. But because it's only six weeks, you can meet your weekly goals and not feel as though it'll be endless. Sure, I could tell you that this book is a "program for life" (snore) and will "change your life" (scary), but I just want you to feel hot and look hotter in your bikini. The fact is that we have zero control over life's snafus, which may explain why the average attrition rate for any fitness program is about 50 percent. So, I've found, in my very long fitness career, short-term goals are much more obtainable and don't set you up for failure. I'd rather you hit it hard for six weeks.

So, commit to The Countdown for six weeks, and I promise to walk you through it, step by step. Sign a contract with yourself to stick with this plan. Put that contract where you will see it every day, and remember that you're only six weeks away from being fearless in your bikini. Don't forget the best part—incentives! When you complete your goals for that week, buy yourself something you've been drooling over, like a sexy pair of Jimmy Choos (I know you're worth it) or a relaxing, tension-ridding massage.

## HOW THE SIX-WEEK PLAN WORKS

If you've been doing the same thing over and over, here's some good news. You're going to put the fun back into your workouts; otherwise, you'll get bored and so will your muscles. In body language: you won't lose weight, you won't find your abs, or worse, those lumps and bumps won't disappear ... aargh. But by doing something totally different, you'll shake and shock those sleepy muscles into bikini shape.

I have created a fitness plan that mixes it up, using my expertise in both fitness and Pilates. The Six-Week Bikini Countdown is the first book to blend traditional fitness with a mind and body workout. The reason? You need it all to have a healthy, sexy body! By learning Pilates, you'll be stronger in your core and more effective in other areas of fitness, such as strength training and cardio—and vice versa. Each week gets increasingly harder, as I give you a whole collection of exercises, including Pilates, to tone your trouble zones (your abs will be sexier than ever) plus fun boot camp and cardio challenges to give you a killer figure.

You'll need some basic equipment; a step platform, and dumbbells and balls in various sizes and weights.

# Take a look at what you'll be doing over the next six weeks:

**week one:**

MONDAY: Burning Fat with Cardio Intervals
TUESDAY: Getting an All Over Makeover
WEDNESDAY: Burning Fat with Cardio Intervals
THURSDAY: Getting Another All Over Makeover
FRIDAY: Burning Fat with Cardio Intervals
SATURDAY: Achieving Lovely Abs with Pilates
SUNDAY: Putting Your (Beautiful) Toes Up

**week two:**

MONDAY: Turning On and Toning Up with Body Boot Camp
TUESDAY: Getting Lean with Cardio
WEDNESDAY: Using Pilates for a Speedy Butt Lift
THURSDAY: Turning On and Toning Up with Body Boot Camp
FRIDAY: Getting Lean with Cardio
SATURDAY: Using Pilates for a Speedy Butt Lift
SUNDAY: Letting Go!

**week three:**

MONDAY: Meeting the Cardio Challenge
TUESDAY: Getting an All Over Hard-Core Workout
WEDNESDAY: Meeting the Cardio Challenge
THURSDAY: Getting an All Over Hard-Core Workout
FRIDAY: Meeting the Cardio Challenge
SATURDAY: Showing Off Simply Gorgeous Abs with Pilates
SUNDAY: Taking It Easy–You're Worth It!

**week four:**

MONDAY: Burning It Off with Boot-Camp-Strength Intervals
TUESDAY: Stepping on It with Steady-State Cardio
WEDNESDAY: Lifting Your Bottom Line with Pilates
THURSDAY: Burning It Off with Boot-Camp-Strength Intervals
FRIDAY: Stepping on It with Steady-State Cardio
SATURDAY: Lifting Your Bottom Line with Pilates
SUNDAY: Enjoying Yourself!

**week five:**

MONDAY: Fighting Fat Faster with Cardio
TUESDAY: Achieving an All Over Balance Workout
WEDNESDAY: Fighting Fat Faster with Cardio
THURSDAY: Achieving an All Over Balance Workout
FRIDAY: Fighting Fat Faster with Cardio
SATURDAY: Sculpting Beach-Worthy Abs: Pilates with Props
SUNDAY: Being Lazy!

**week six:**

MONDAY: Becoming Fabulous with Boot-Camp-Strength Intervals
TUESDAY: Getting Bikini Lean with Steady-State Cardio
WEDNESDAY: Busting Your Booty with Pilates
THURSDAY: Becoming Fabulous with Boot-Camp-Strength Intervals
FRIDAY: Getting Bikini Lean with Steady State Cardio
SATURDAY: Busting Your Booty with Pilates
SUNDAY: Celebrating You!

Whew! That's a lot. Here's a warning, though: you have to be moderately fit before you begin the program, because within each week, the goals will ramp up to burn calories, build strong muscles (and bones), and keep your heart healthy. The payoff, of course, is a fearless bikini body.

## BIKINI SHOPPING

To hit the beach with bikini confidence you have to uncover the hidden areas of your body. So unless you look forward to spending the summer in a burkatini, I'm going to suggest the unthinkable: go bikini shopping. I get it, you may not be ready to see every dimple or roll, but ignoring your trouble spots won't make them go away. So bare it all and try on lots of bikinis. Pick your favorite one, but don't buy one that breaks the bank, because it isn't going fit you in six weeks. In other words, instead of the scale, this bikini you buy will track your body results. Put it on before you start and then every two weeks and take notes on how you look and feel in your bikini: Are your thighs tighter? Do you feel like you have a little more room in the bottom? What about those dimples and rolls? Get the point? Stay committed, and then say hello to your bikini body.

## PILATES: A STRONG, SEXY SPINE AND THE BEST BIKINI ABS

Bikini abs are made (not born) with Pilates (puh-LAH-teez). Some of the benefits of Pilates include strong muscles, a sexy and flat stomach, a delicious bum, and a taller and tighter appearance. But that's not all. Pilates can help you move more efficiently in both these six weeks and in your everyday life, because each exercise strengthens what Joseph Pilates called your powerhouse or "central girdle of strength," meaning your abdominal, back, and hip muscles. The secret to a sexy, strong spine is a ninety-year-old method that gently stretches and strengthens your ab and back muscles.

Your spine is your life support and consists of a complex system of bones, ligaments, muscles, and nerves, while your postural muscles (your abdominal, back, and pelvic floor) form an internal girdle to stabilize and support your spine. Strengthen these muscles, and you're on your way to a sexy, strong spine. That's where Pilates comes in. Not only will you strengthen your powerhouse, but you'll also focus on keeping your spinal bones aligned and healthy.

Sexy backs have three natural curves: the first is the slight curve in your neck called the cervical spine, making up the first seven vertebrae; the second is the middle back or thoracic spine, which is slightly extended and adds up to twelve vertebrae; and finally, the third is between the pelvis and the spine, which is the lumbar spine or lower back. Your spine has two fused bones acting as one unit: five sacral vertebrae make up the flat bone of the sacrum, and the coccygeal vertebrae are the nonmovable bones of your tailbone.

Poor posture is not sexy and not healthy! A potbelly isn't sexy, pain can leave you feeling anything but sexy, and slouchy shoulders can shorten you an inch or more–so not sexy. The truth is, if you don't train your muscles to support a strong spine and be aware of your posture throughout your day, over time you can change the way you look, leaving you not so sexy in your bikini! There isn't an exercise program out there that shapes your abs like Pilates. It will get you bikini-ready from the inside and out, so it helps to know a little about the muscles that keep your spine strong.

### THE SIX GUIDING PRINCIPLES OF PILATES

To get your best bikini body, use these six guiding principles:

**Concentrate:** Think before you move your body; it's the will of your mind that tells your body what to do.

**Control:** Move with control; no jerks. If you don't move with control, you may injure yourself.

**Center:** Every move begins from your center, including your spine and its surrounding muscles. A strong core can better support movement from your arms and legs.

**Flow:** Each move flows from one to another as if in a beautiful dance.

**Precision:** Make it look easy; each move is done with precision and control.

**Breathe:** Breath work is at the heart of each Pilates exercise. Each move is coordinated with movement so the body and breath flow as one. The breath work in Pilates is totally different than everyday breathing. You'll breathe into your rib cage, expanding your ribs as if an inner tube were opening your rib cage, and then exhale deeply, as if you were wringing out a dirty sponge, to close your rib cage. Inhale through the nose and then exhale through the mouth. Try it!

### POSITIONING YOUR FEET: THE PILATES "V"

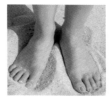

You'll always work in a foot position called a Pilates "V," meaning the heels of your feet touch as your toes open about three fingers' width apart. This slight turnout engages your inner thigh muscles and pelvic floor. Squeeze, squeeze, and squeeze for sexier inner thighs and lift, lift, and lift through your pelvic floor, or imagine your bladder is full and a restroom in nowhere in sight!

### THE TECHNIQUE

Starting position: In a standing position, put your heels together and open your toes about three fingers' width apart. Squeeze your inner thighs to get a "wrap feeling."

### TIPS AND TRICKS

- Place a rolled-up hand towel between your legs to help you engage your inner thighs.
- If you have back issues or are bowlegged, for example, stay on the safe side and work with your feet parallel to each other or with your big toes touching so as not to aggravate your back. Check with your doctor.

## KEEPING YOUR BEAUTIFUL SPINE NEUTRAL

While doing Pilates pay attention to how you're moving your pelvis, because its position affects your lower back, or lumbar spine curve. As you go through these six weeks, keep in mind that your body is a closed-chain system, meaning that what happens in one part of the body will eventually affect another part. Because your pelvis attaches your legs to your spine, it takes a pounding when you run, walk, or jump, and it absorbs stress from your body when, for example, you carry something really heavy. To minimize stress on your body, your pelvis must stabilize itself so your lumbar spine does not take on needless stress. This stabilizing position is called a neutral pelvis, which is one component of a neutral spine (also called "good posture"), meaning your bones, ligaments, muscles, and discs are aligned.

When doing the Pilates exercises over the next six weeks, you'll set up each exercise with good body alignment, because this puts the least amount of stress on your body as you move it, while also strengthening the muscles that reinforce good posture. You'll also use your pelvis as your first point of reference. If you're holding your pelvis incorrectly, you may feel the stress in your lower back; over time, you may even alter the bones of your spine!

FINDING NEUTRAL: Moving your pelvis in and out of neutral

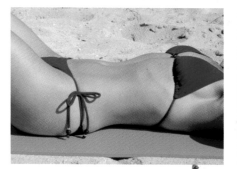

Your lower back is just right (neutral pelvis)

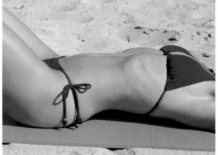

Your lower back has too much arch (anterior tilt)

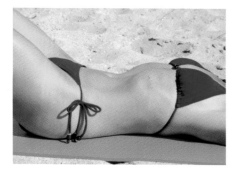

Your lower back is too flat (posterior tilt)

## SEXY TO YOUR CORE

In Pilates, you'll move your spine in all of its natural movements: forward bend (flexion) and backward bend (extension), twist right and left (rotation), and reach from side to side (side bend). To do this, you need strength from a variety of muscles, including your hips, abs, and back. These core muscles wrap around your center and are made up of layers and layers of muscles to support, stabilize, and move your spine. Think of an onion, peel away each layer of skin and eventually you get to its soft spine. Well, your body is no different.

Pilates takes inches off your waist because every exercise works your core and mainly focuses on strengthening your abdominal muscles as a group. Take a look at the following illustration to get a glimpse of your abs.

**1.** Your deepest abdominal muscle forms an internal girdle for your center; it's called the transversus abdominis, or transverse. In Pilates, you'll exhale deeply to engage this muscle because it provides a girdle of support for your lumber spine by literally wrapping low around your waist. As you practice and get stronger, you can actually feel this contraction in your lower belly, tightening from hip bone to hip bone and lifting your pubic bone to your belly button. Think of zipping up your favorite pair of skinny jeans to feel your lower belly.

**2.** Sitting on top of your transverse are your obliques; internal obliques sit deep and rest on top of your transverse, while external obliques are superficial. Between the two, they help support your center and let you twist and bend sideways at the waist.

**3.** The most superficial of the group is the rectus abdominis, the long muscle extending from your pubic bone to your sternum. This muscle lets you bend forward at the waist and compresses your rib cage. When these muscles are strong as a group, your body works better, looks sexier, and can protect your spine from injury.

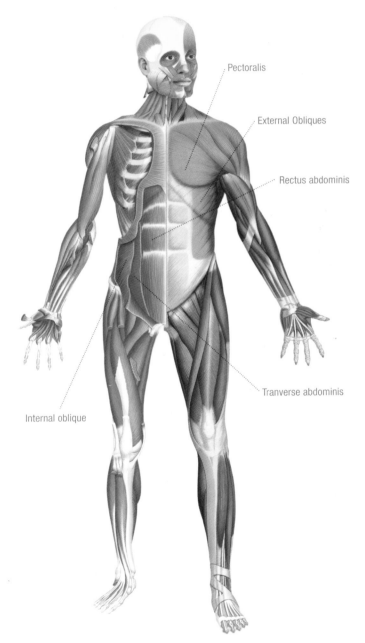

Pectoralis

External Obliques

Rectus abdominis

Tranverse abdominis

Internal oblique

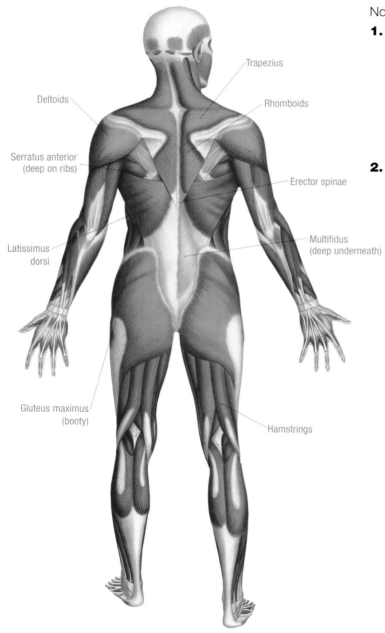

Trapezius

Deltoids

Rhomboids

Serratus anterior
(deep on ribs)

Erector spinae

Latissimus
dorsi

Multifidus
(deep underneath)

Gluteus maximus
(booty)

Hamstrings

Now look at your back muscles.

**1.** Strong back muscles are sexy, too. Your deepest back muscle, called the multifidus, works around the clock to stabilize and support your spine. Because it extends from the sacrum to the cervical vertebrae and provides three layers of protection for your spine, it works overtime to keep your back healthy and fit while assisting in moving the spine in extension (arching) and rotation (twisting).

**2.** Sitting on top of your multifidus are your erector spinae, or spinal erectors. Collectively, these muscles run from the sacrum to the last two thoracic vertebrae and help keep your back straight (honoring the natural curves) with perfect posture. Just about every exercise or sport calls on these muscles, so again, it's important to keep them fit and strong. Lastly, your pelvic floor makes up your bottom core; these muscles also assist in spinal and pelvic stability. Collectively, your pelvic floor makes a sling or hammock of muscles that attaches in two different directions, from your pubic bone and tailbone, and from one butt bone to another to support the weight of your organs. To engage these muscles, think of an elevator: on the ground floor your pelvic floor is relaxed; push the button and the elevator will travel up to the first floor. In your body, exhale to lift your pelvic floor deep into your center. Here's the trick, pretend that you have to go to the bathroom and there's not a bathroom in sight! Collectively, these muscles move the bones of your pelvis and help stabilize it. What's important is to engage deep within your center, lifting from your pelvic floor while your belly button moves toward your spine. Remember to keep your belly button toward your spine the entire time.

## SEXY SHOULDERS

You can look sexier and taller just by standing up straight, which is why Pilates is said to "lengthen" your muscles, when in fact it actually strengthens the muscles that support good posture. And like your pelvis, your shoulder girdle attaches your arms to your spine and absorbs the stress of your arms. Anything you carry, groceries, children, a laptop, is better supported by strong upper back muscles and a fit spine.

In Pilates, you'll strengthen the muscles of your upper back: middle back (thoracic) and neck (cervical) to support a healthy posture. To do this, you'll stabilize your shoulder blades, the two winged bones on your upper spine. Try this, lift your shoulders to your ears and slightly back, and then slide your shoulder blades down your back and don't move them. With this, you may feel a little taller and perhaps your chest opens up. Imagine that you have a set of deep pockets resting on your upper back ready for your shoulder blades. Throughout the next six weeks, you'll hear me say "pits to hips," and this is what I mean. Like your pelvis, your shoulder blades are another point of reference, because their position can also affect the posture of your upper back and neck. Working with, for example, your shoulders lifted toward your ears can injure the very delicate muscles on your upper back. Over time, this changes the way you look and may even create a downward cycle of aches and pains.

Take a look at the muscles of your upper back:

1. Moving your shoulders in all directions requires a variety of muscles. Some of the heavy hitters are your trapezius, or traps, which form a diamond-shaped muscle originating on the base of the skull, attaching the shoulder blades and ending around the middle of your back; it's your traps that assist in lowering and lifting your shoulders.

2. Sitting between your shoulder blades are the rhomboids, which help stabilize your shoulder blades and draw your shoulder blades together to open your chest.

3. Then there is the serratus anterior, which is a thin muscle that originates on your lateral ribs and connects under your shoulder blades. This muscle, too, helps stabilize your shoulder blades to keep them flat on your back while keeping your shoulders in place.

4. The biggest back muscle is the latissimus dorsi, or lats; it fans across your back and extends from the lower spine to the upper arm bone.

5. And then, there are your deltoids, which are your shoulder muscles. They blanket your shoulders and are comprised of the anterior, middle, and posterior deltoids; these muscles help move your arms in various positions.

6. On the front of your body are your pectorals, which form a broad band of chest muscles.

When strong, all the postural muscles work in harmony to enhance your figure. As you move along through these next six weeks, pay attention to how you're holding your upper spine. Pilates can help you move more efficiently in general, and it especially builds spinal strength to support an active body.

## CHIN TO CHEST

Your head is an extension of your spine, and many Pilates exercises require you to curl up and hold your chin to your chest. To work your abs (and protect your neck), imagine you are holding an egg between your chin and your chest. If you don't have the abdominal strength, then it may be hard to hold this position. So please don't struggle to hold your head up, because you may injure the many delicate muscles that make up your neck spine. Instead, rest your head on the mat, and then try the exercise again after a short break. Also, always think about the spine as a whole and your head is just part of it. In Pilates terms: "head in line with your spine."

It's important to approach your head and neck with great respect, because these muscles, soft tissues, and bones are delicate. Never jerk your head around, and always think about proper alignment while you're on the treadmill, lifting weights, or doing Pilates.

With good posture, your neck spine should have a slight exaggeration, but I've seen chronic tightness alter this connection, leaving a variety of muscle groups weak in the process. Still, neck issues can originate from another part of the spine, osteoporosis is a good example. Remember, what happens in one part of the spine will eventually affect another part. So please pay attention to your spine at all times. A sexy, healthy spine is worth all the trouble even in these early stages. Joseph Pilates said, "You're as old as your spine is flexible."

## CARDIO: YOUR BIKINI BODY IN MOTION

The fastest way to melt the fat and burn the calories is by adding high-intensity bursts to your cardio workouts. In the next six weeks, you'll see two different cardio workouts: either kicking it into high gear with cardio intervals or doing some nice and easy cardio days. Why? Because it's the fastest way to your bikini body!

So follow the weekly workout routine discussed in the "How the Six-Week Plan Works" section earlier in this introduction. Even better, you can photocopy it and hang it on your refrigerator for a quick reference. All cardio workouts in this book are listed in terms of walking and/or running on a treadmill. If you prefer other cardio machines: stair stepper, elliptical trainer, stationary bike, rowing machine or non-machine cardio workouts, outdoor walking, running, swimming, use the following perceived exertion scale to monitor how hard you're working during your cardio workouts.

0    Bed rest
1    Watching television
2    Getting up to make popcorn
3    Slow walk
4    Walk
5    Brisk walk; your breathing is slightly elevated
6    Light exercise; you're breathing hard but you can carry on a conversation

## PILATES HAS A LANGUAGE ALL ITS OWN

Keep the following terminology in mind as you practice Pilates:

**Belly button to spine:** Move your belly button up and under your ribs and back to your spine to engage your lower belly and support your lower back.

**Pits to hips:** Engage your upper back muscles by dropping your shoulders back and down before you move.

**Chin to chest:** Look between your legs and imagine an egg rests between your chin and chest.

**Lift through your center:** Lift your pelvic floor up to get extra work and power.

**Breathe:** Inhale through the nose and then exhale through the mouth.

**Back flat on mat:** When your legs are up at ninety degrees or lower, say your toes are in line with your nose, your back may arch from the mat. Engage your abs to work in a neutral position while protecting your lower back.

**Scoop your abs:** Engaging your abs, create a scoop in your belly as if scooping out your abs, your belly will hollow. No bulgy belly or loaf of bread in your belly. I'll say this tons of times during the next six weeks, but that's how you'll get those bikini abs!

7   Vigorous exercise; breathless; it's hard to talk normally
8   Very vigorous exercise; choppy words; you can spit out a word or two
9   Intense exercise; can't talk while exercising
10  All out sprint

Your goal is to alternate between a steady pace and a run, working between levels 5 and 6 and at times going between 7 and 9. You should be breathing hard and able to talk normally in recovery, and then experience breathless to choppy to can't talk while going all out. Sweat can also be a good indication that you're working hard enough. If you're not sweating, increase your intensity.

One word of caution: depending on the manufacturer, cardio machines may vary, so you have to experiment with intensity and incline levels even on a treadmill. Even though I have given you routine guidelines for the treadmill, use the preceding intensity scale to dictate how hard you're working. During all the cardio interval workouts in this book, you won't be able to read your favorite magazine or even read the news scroll on TV.

## STRENGTH TRAINING: DEFINING YOUR BIKINI BODY

Strength training is normally not a huge calorie blaster, but it can be if you pick up the pace with strength training intervals. So you'll get sexy muscles with two different workouts over the next six weeks: "all over makeovers" will sculpt your muscles while the "boot camp" workouts will scorch the calories and give you cardio benefits.
Depending on the week, you'll do one or the other, so follow the six-week workout plan, and soon you'll say, "Hello, bikini."

You'll see the terms "sets" and "reps" (or "repetitions") during the next six weeks. "Reps" defines how many times you need to do an exercise, while a "set" refers to the series of exercises.

Always do a five-minute warm-up before each strength training session–walking is a great warm-up!

## EATING YOUR WAY TO A BIKINI BODY

In the end, it's all about calories in versus calories out, so although every workout is designed to burn mega calories, you have to do your part and eat right. No amount of exercise can repair the damage caused by overeating or eating the wrong foods. So in each of the "Sunday" sections throughout this book, you'll find a few of my favorite tips to help you get your bikini bod ready!

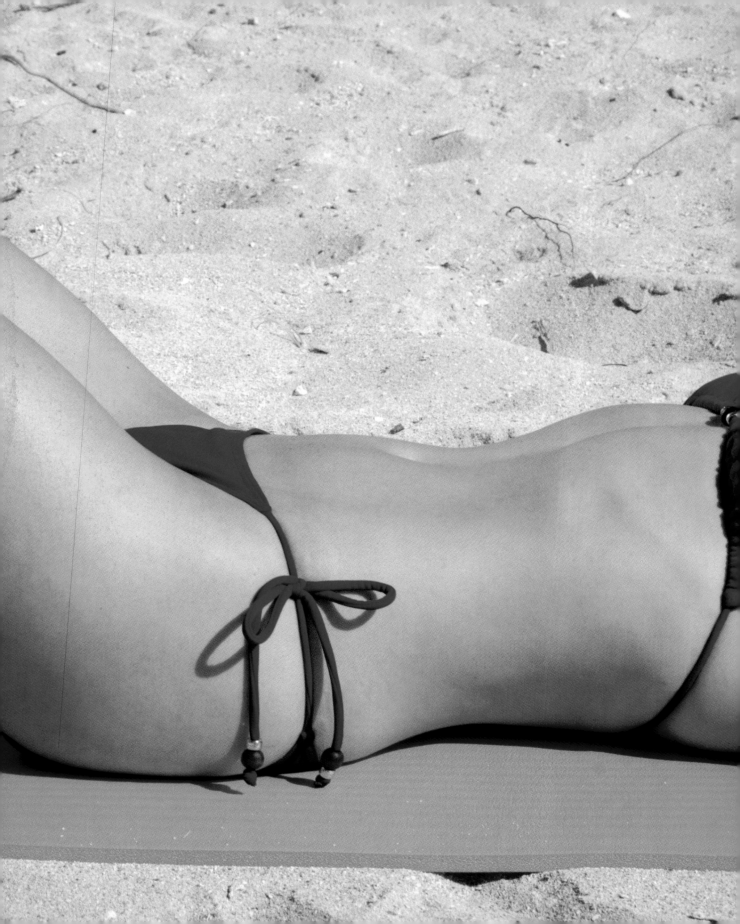

## BIKINI BODY BLAST OFF

So you want to feel gutsy on the beach without a sarong covering your bottom, but you're not sure where to begin. That's easy—your bikini body blast off begins by blitzing some mega calories. This week, your goal is to burn, baby, burn those calories with lots of cardio. Don't worry you won't be spending hours at the gym. Instead you'll make each workout count in a huge way. Your target calorie burn for each workout will hit around 500 sweaty unwanted calories. The payoff, of course, is that *itsy-bitsy bikini.*

| | |
|---|---|
| **MONDAY** | Burning Fat with Cardio Intervals |
| **TUESDAY** | Getting an All Over Makeover |
| **WEDNESDAY** | Burning Fat with Cardio Intervals |
| **THURSDAY** | Getting Another All Over Makeover |
| **FRIDAY** | Burning Fat with Cardio Intervals |
| **SATURDAY** | Achieving Lovely Abs with Pilates |
| **SUNDAY** | Putting Your (Beautiful) Toes Up |

# WORKOUT PROGRAM AT A GLANCE

|  |  |  |  |
|---|---|---|---|
| **MONDAY** | **TUESDAY** | **WEDNESDAY** | **THURSDAY** |
| Burning Fat with Cardio Intervals | Getting an All Over Makeover | Burning Fat with Cardio Intervals | Getting Another All Over Makeover |

**MONDAY**

**Burning Fat with Cardio Intervals**

1. 3 minutes: Warm up by walking 3.2 mph (5.1 kph), no grade
2. 8 minutes: Walk 3.5 to 4 mph (5.5 to 6.1 kph), no grade
3. 2 minutes: Run 5 to 6 mph (8.1 to 9.5 kph), no grade
4. Repeat steps 2 and 3 four more times
5. 2 minutes: Cool down by walking 2.5 to 3 mph (4.0 to 4.5 kph), no grade

**TUESDAY**

**Getting an All Over Makeover**

**SET 1**

Squat with Dumbbells
3 sets of 15 to 20 reps

Chest Press
3 sets of 15 to 20 reps

Triceps Kickbacks
3 sets of 15 to 20 reps

**SET 2**

Reverse Lunge with Dumbbells
3 sets of 15 to 20 reps

Bent Over Row
3 sets of 15 to 20 reps

Biceps Curls
3 sets of 15 to 20 reps

**SET 3**

Deadlift with Dumbbells
3 sets of 15 to 20 reps

Reverse Fly
3 sets of 15 to 20 reps

Side Arm Raise
3 sets of 15 to 20 reps

Front Arm Raise
3 sets of 15 to 20 reps

**WEDNESDAY**

**Burning Fat with Cardio Intervals**

1. 3 minutes: Warm up by walking 3.2 mph (5.1 kph), no grade
2. 8 minutes: Walk 3.5 to 4 mph (5.5 to 6.1 kph), no grade
3. 2 minutes: Run 5 to 6 mph (8.1 to 9.5 kph), no grade
4. Repeat steps 2 and 3 four more times
5. 2 minutes: Cool down by walking 2.5 to 3 mph (4.0 to 4.5 kph), no grade

**THURSDAY**

**Getting Another All Over Makeover**

**SET 1**

Squat with Dumbbells
3 sets of 15 to 20 reps

Chest Press
3 sets of 15 to 20 reps

Triceps Kickbacks
3 sets of 15 to 20 reps

**SET 2**

Reverse Lunge with Dumbbells
3 sets of 15 to 20 reps

Bent Over Row
3 sets of 15 to 20 reps

Biceps Curls
3 sets of 15 to 20 reps

**SET 3**

Deadlift with Dumbbells
3 sets of 15 to 20 reps

Reverse Fly
3 sets of 15 to 20 reps

Side Arm Raise
3 sets of 15 to 20 reps

Front Arm Raise
3 sets of 15 to 20 reps

| **FRIDAY** | **SATURDAY** | **SUNDAY** |
|---|---|---|

## Burning Fat with Cardio Intervals

## Achieving Lovely Abs with Pilates

## Putting Your (Beautiful) Toes Up

OFF

1. 3 minutes: Warm up by walking 3.2 mph (5.1 kph), no grade

2. 8 minutes: Walk 3.5 to 4 mph (5.5 to 6.1 kph), no grade

3. 2 minutes: Run 5 to 6 mph (8.1 to 9.5 kph), no grade

4. Repeat steps 2 and 3 four more times

5. 2 minutes: Cool down by walking 2.5 to 3 mph (4.0 to 4.5 kph), no grade

**The following are the Pilates exercises you'll be doing today:**

The Hundred

Roll-up

Single Leg Circle

Rolling Like a Ball

Single Leg Stretch

Double Leg Stretch

Spine Stretch

Corkscrew

Saw

Swan

Child's Pose

Single Leg Kick

Shoulder Bridge

Teaser 1

The Seal

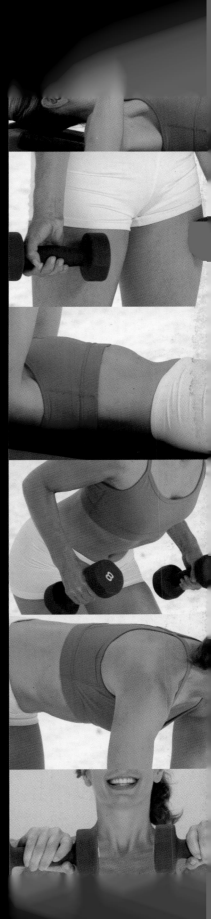

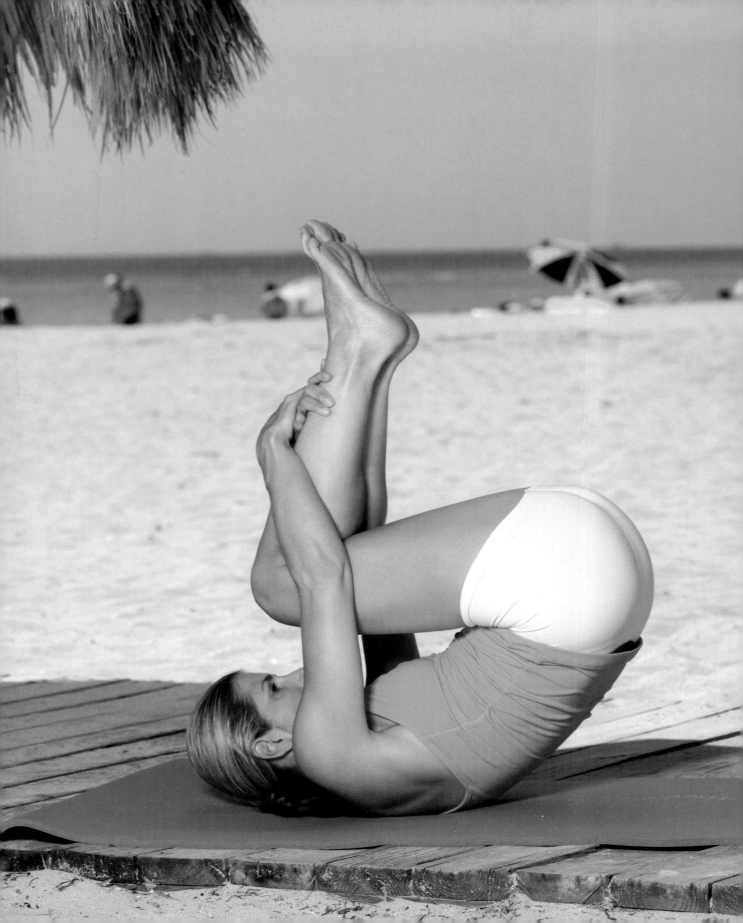

# MONDAY: BURNING FAT WITH CARDIO INTERVALS

According to a new study from the University of Guelph in Ontario, Jason Talanian, Ph.D., found that interval training burns more fat and increases fitness more quickly than constant, but moderately intense, physical activity.

A study from the University of New South Wales in Sydney echoes these findings: women who spent 20 minutes cycling, rotating high and low-intensity intervals, lost three times the fat off their legs and butt in 15 weeks than women who exercised at a continuous, regular pace for 40 minutes.

For this reason, you're going to do intervals today! Leave the magazine at home because it will only get sticky and wet. It's time to hit the treadmill and do a cardio interval session. To burn mega calories, you'll alternate between high- (running) and low-intensity (power walking) intervals to keep your heart rate high. If you don't have a gym membership or you get bored with treadmills, do this workout outside and make friends with the wind and hills. For added intensity, simply look for a hill on which you can do the intervals that are on a grade. If you prefer to use other cardio equipment (stationary bike, elliptical trainer, stair stepper, and so on), or you want to walk and run outside, check out the introduction to this book for tips on how to gauge your intensity levels. Your cardio sessions will last 50 to 55 minutes, including a warm-up and a cool down. (Note: "grade" refers to the amount of incline you set on your treadmill.)

The following is your workout:

1. 3 minutes: Warm up by walking 3.2 mph (5.1 kph), no grade
2. 8 minutes: Walk 3.5 to 4 mph (5.5 to 6.1 kph), no grade
3. 2 minutes: Run 5 to 6 mph (8.1 to 9.5 kph), no grade
4. Repeat steps 2 and 3 four more times
5. 2 minutes: Cool down by walking 2.5 to 3 mph (4.0 to 4.5 kph), no grade

If you don't have a treadmill, pick another cardio machine: stair stepper, elliptical trainer, or a stationary bike. Mixing it up can also save you from an injury because you're not doing the same old stuff! Don't forget to alternate between low- and high-intensity levels. Use the treadmill workout from Fat Burning Workout #1 as your guide.

# TUESDAY: GETTING AN ALL OVER MAKEOVER

On Tuesday, you'll do a 45-minute to 1-hour strength session, which you'll repeat on Thursday. This is a fairly easy all over workout because these exercises are the foundation of the more intense exercises in the remaining chapters of this book. What's most important is your alignment, which is why each exercise has accompanying tips and tricks to make sure you're doing the exercises correctly.

To get the most from the workout, keep moving at a fairly nice pace, without stopping frequently to rest. Move from one exercise right into the next. If you start to feel your form deteriorating because of fatigue, do take a short break. Before each strength or cardio workout, include a 5-minute warm-up on a cardio machine, such as walking 3.2 to 3.5 mph/ 5.0 to 5.6 kph on a treadmill.

You'll need a couple sets of dumbbells. For your legs and butt, the dumbbells need to be heavy enough to finish a set with good form, which is 15 to 20 pounds (7 to 9 kg) for most women. For your arms, use a lighter pair of dumbbells, 8 to 10 pounds (4 to 5 kg).

To do this all over workout you'll do each of the three exercises in Set 1, doing 15 to 20 reps of each, and then you'll do the three exercises in Set 1 two more times. For example, you'll complete 15 to 20 slow and controlled reps of each of the following exercises: Squat with Dumbbells, Chest Press, and Triceps Kickbacks. Repeat that set two times before doing the same with Set 2, and then finishing with Set 3. Total time should be about 45 minutes to 1 hour. If you're not clear on what a set or a rep is, flip to the introduction section of this book.

**SET 1**

Squat with Dumbbells
  3 sets of 15 to 20 reps

Chest Press
  3 sets of 15 to 20 reps

Triceps Kickbacks
  3 sets of 15 to 20 reps

**SET 2**

Reverse Lunge with Dumbbells
  3 sets of 15 to 20 reps

Bent Over Row
  3 sets of 15 to 20 reps

Biceps Curls
  3 sets of 15 to 20 reps

**SET 3**

Deadlift with Dumbbells
  3 sets of 15 to 20 reps

Reverse Fly
  3 sets of 15 to 20 reps

Side Arm Raise
  3 sets of 15 to 20 reps

Front Arm Raise
  3 sets of 15 to 20 reps

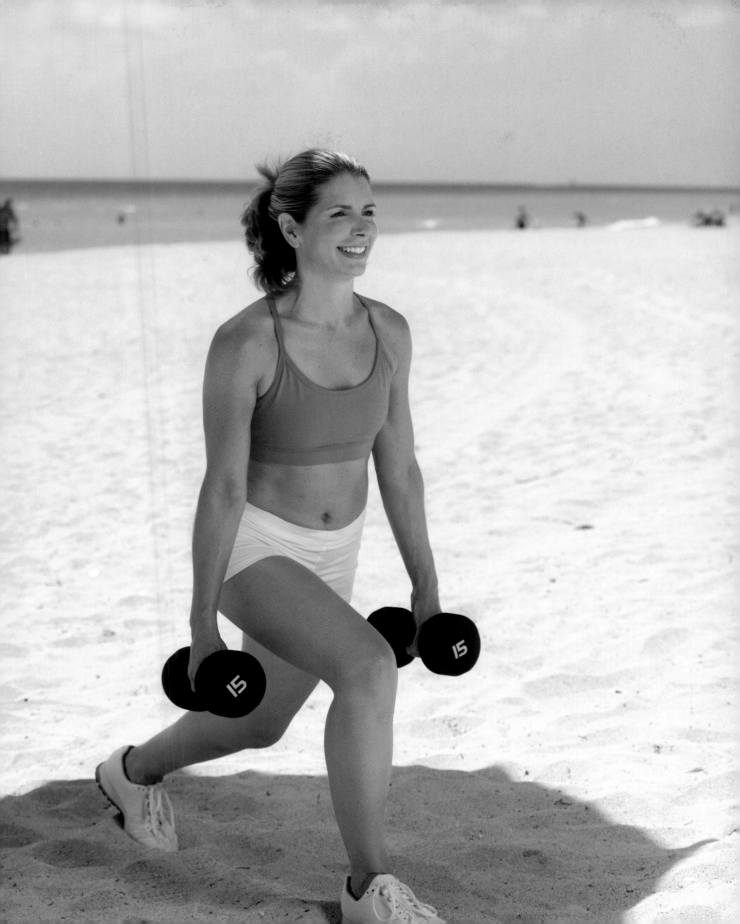

# Squat with Dumbbells

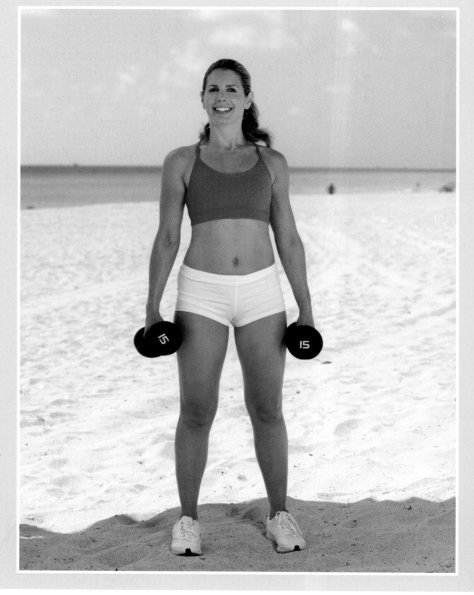

**STARTING POSITION:** Stand with your feet a little wider than hip width apart and grasp a 15- to 20-pound (7 to 9 kg) dumbbell in each hand. Look forward and slightly up.

**TIPS AND TRICKS**

- Don't lean forward; your torso will naturally come forward slightly as you squat.

- Don't turn your knees in; keep your knees stable and point your toes forward as you squat down.

- Use sexy posture; straighten your spine from the top of your head down and relax your shoulders.

- Don't overarch your lower back; turn on your abs to provide support for your lower back.

- If you want extra butt work, sit back on your heels so your hips and knees are parallel to the floor. Also, try sitting on the end of a bench to make sure your butt bones touch at the same time to ensure you are using your muscles evenly.

# THE PAYOFF:

Gives you a booty makeover.

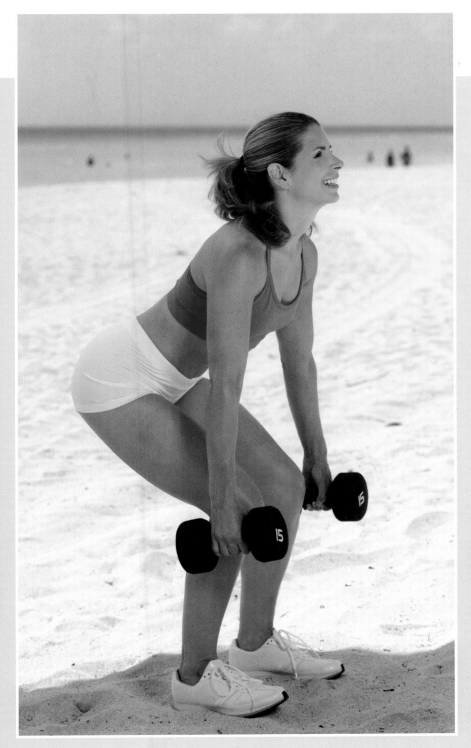

**POSITION 1:** Lower your booty until your thighs are parallel to the floor, knees aligned with your second and third toes. Keep your chest lifted and your spine straight as you imagine sitting your booty in a chair. Do 15 to 20 reps.

# Chest Press

REPLAY WEEK TWO

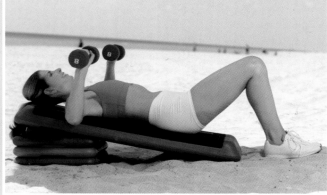

**STARTING POSITION:** Using 8- to 10-pound (4 to 5 kg) dumbbells, lie flat on your back, either on the bench or a step. Lower your arms out to the sides until your elbows are in line with your shoulders so you can see the weights in your peripheral vision. You may feel a slight stretch in the chest area.

### TIPS AND TRICKS

- Don't swing your arms; use control to lift and lower your weights.
- Don't lift your lower back off the bench; engage your abs to support your lower back. If you can't stabilize your torso, drop down in weight; your weights may be too heavy.

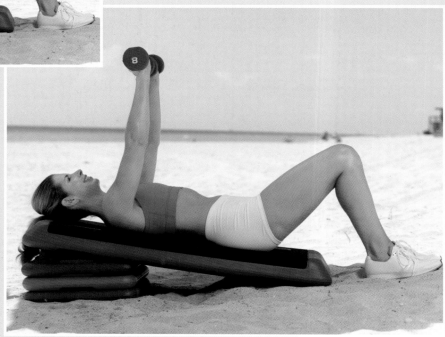

**POSITION 1:** Raise your arms up and together. Pause, and then slowly lower your arms. Do 15 to 20 reps.

## THE PAYOFF:

Develops stunning, sexy, and strong chest.

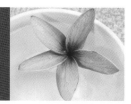

# Triceps Kickbacks

REPLAY WEEK TWO

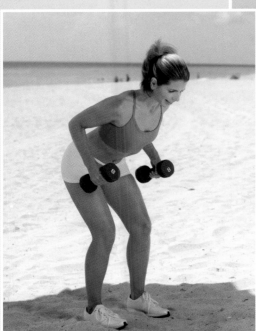

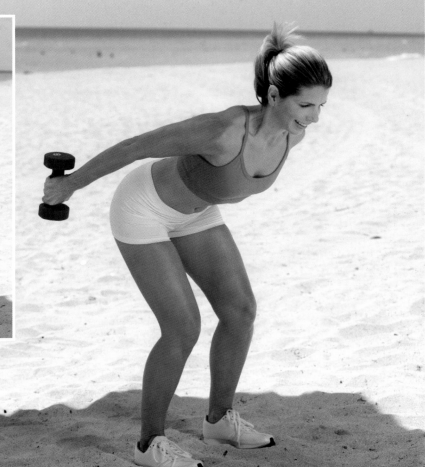

**STARTING POSITION:** Stand in a squat position with an 8- to 10-pound (4 to 5 kg) dumbbell in each hand, knees slightly bent and feet hip width apart. Bend over so that your back is almost parallel to the ground. Bend your elbows to about 90 degrees, raising them to just above your back.

### TIPS AND TRICKS

- Don't round your spine; keep your abs active and lengthen from the top of your head.

**POSITION 1:** Straighten your arms backward, leading with your pinky finger. Keep your upper arms stationary and near your ribs. When they're fully extended, your arms should be parallel to the ground. Do 15 to 20 reps.

## THE PAYOFF:

Eliminates flabby arms.

# Reverse Lunge with Dumbbells

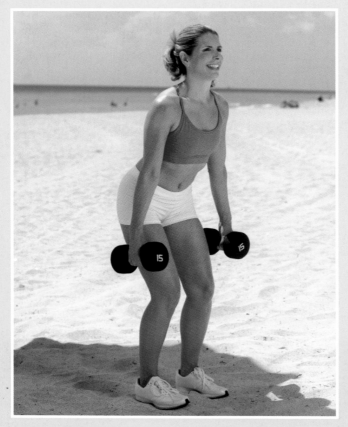

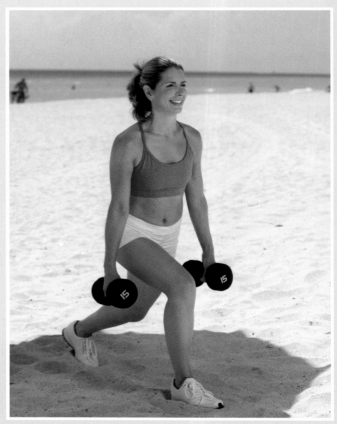

**STARTING POSITION:** Stand with your legs together, bend your knees and slightly lean forward. Hold your 15- to 20-pound (7 to 9 kg) dumbbells in your hands and straighten your arms by your sides.

**POSITION 1:** Lift your right knee and slowly move your left leg behind you as your right leg bends into a lunge position. Repeat on the left side. Do 15 to 20 reps.

**TIPS AND TRICKS**

- Don't lean forward too much; the majority of your body weight is in the lunge leg.
- Don't forget to engage your abs to help keep you steady.

## THE PAYOFF:

Gives you a booty makeover and lean legs.

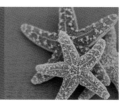

# Bent Over Row

REPLAY WEEK TWO

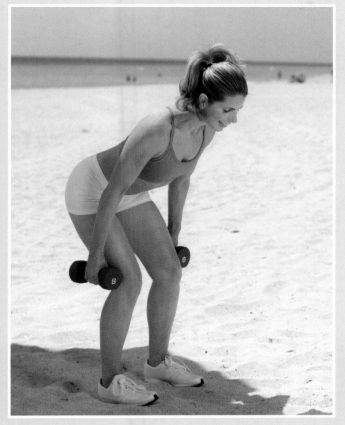

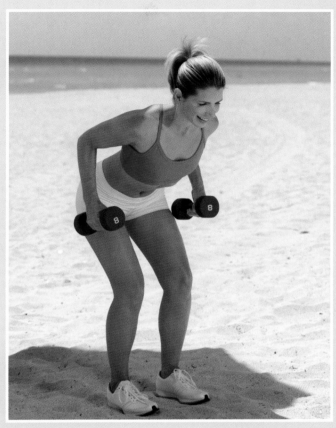

**STARTING POSITION:** Stand with your knees slightly bent and your feet hip width apart. Hold an 8- to 10-pound (4 to 5 kg) dumbbell in each hand and bend from the waist so your back is almost parallel to the floor. Straighten your arms to the floor, palms facing in.

**TIPS AND TRICKS**

- Don't swing your arms; move with control as your knuckles face out, and keep your elbows in line with your shoulders.

**POSITION 1:** Bend your elbows to lift your dumbbells to the ceiling. The dumbbells will slide on the outside of your chest. Pause and return to the starting position. Do 15 to 20 reps.

## THE PAYOFF:

Sculpts a stunning upper back and strong shoulders.

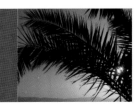

# Biceps Curls

REPLAY WEEK TWO

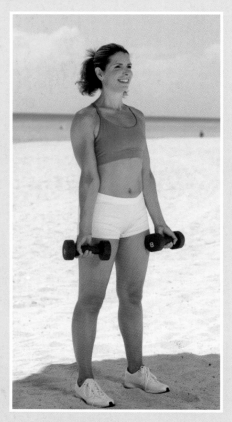

**STARTING POSITION:** Stand with feet hip width apart and hold an 8- to 10-pound (4 to 5 kg) dumbbell in each hand, palms facing up. Straighten your arms so the dumbbells rest just outside of your thighs.

**TIPS AND TRICKS**

- Don't swing your arms as you curl the weight toward your chest.

**POSITION 1:** Keep your elbows close to your torso and curl the dumbbells toward your chest. Do 15 to 20 reps.

## THE PAYOFF:

Overhauls your butt, legs, and core.

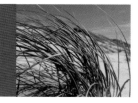

# Deadlift with Dumbbells

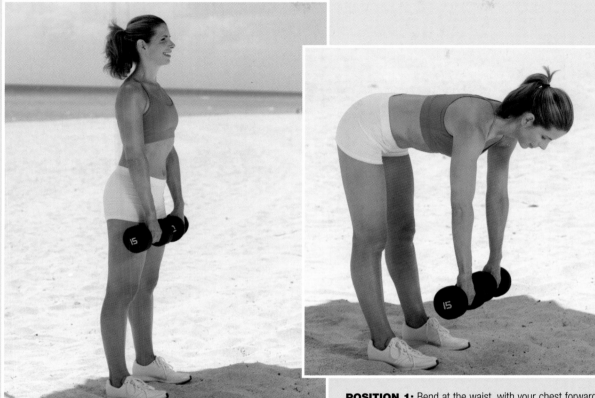

**STARTING POSITION:** Stand with feet hip width apart, with your knees straight. Hold a 15- to 20-pound (7 to 9 kg) dumbbell in each hand.

**POSITION 1:** Bend at the waist, with your chest forward, and keep your legs straight. Lift your navel toward your spine to support your lower back as you return to the starting position. Do 15 to 20 reps.

### TIPS AND TRICKS

- Don't round your spine; keep your torso straight and your head in line with your spine.
- Don't do this exercise if you have a lower back injury; check with your doctor.
- Don't hang in your lower back; engage your abs by lifting your belly button toward your spine, giving your lower back support.

## THE PAYOFF:

Makes for an eye-catching backside and a strong, fit back.

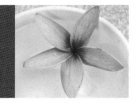

# Reverse Fly

## REPLAY WEEK TWO

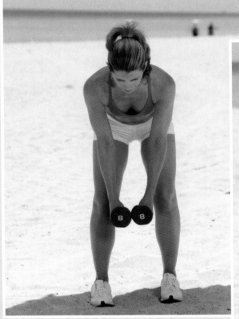

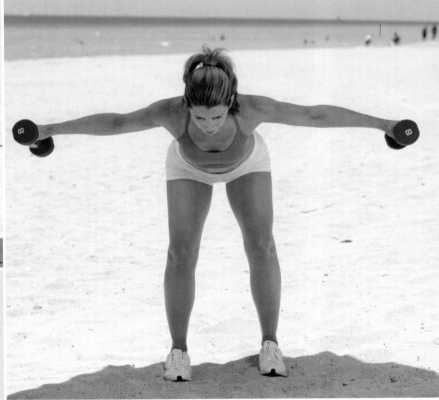

**STARTING POSITION:** Stand with feet hip width apart and in a squat position. Hold an 8- to 10-pound (4 to 5 kg) dumbbell in each hand and bend over from the waist. Turn on your abs to support your lower back. Hang your arms in front, knuckles out, in line with your shoulders.

### TIPS AND TRICKS

- Don't round your shoulders forward; keep your chest lifted and your shoulders back.
- Don't lift your arms higher than your shoulders; engage your upper back muscles to crack a walnut between your shoulder blades—well, at least imagine it!
- Don't swing your arms; move with control.

**POSITION 1:** Lift your arms up and out to the sides of your body until shoulder height, bringing your shoulder blades together. Your elbows are slightly bent. Do 15 to 20 reps.

## THE PAYOFF:

Gives you a super sexy upper back and strong shoulders.

# Side Arm Raise

REPLAY WEEK TWO

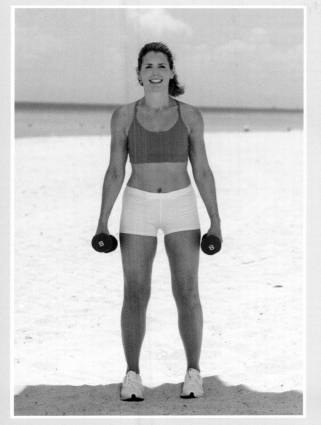

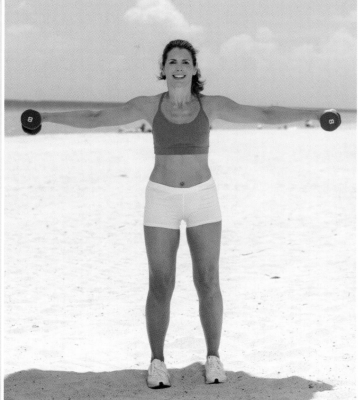

**STARTING POSITION:** Stand with feet hip width apart with soft knees. Hold an 8- to 10-pound (4 to 5 kg) dumbbell in each hand, knuckles face up. Straighten your arms so the dumbbells touch the sides of your thighs, thumbs point in.

**TIPS AND TRICKS**

- Don't bend your wrists; maintain strong arms.
- Don't lift your shoulders to your ears; use your shoulder muscles to lift the arms, not your delicate shoulder joints.

**POSITION 1:** Lift your arms straight out to the sides so the dumbbells end up just below your shoulders. Pause, then return to the starting position. Do 15 to 20 reps.

# THE PAYOFF:

Sculpts strong shoulders.

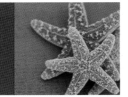

# Front Arm Raise

REPLAY WEEK TWO

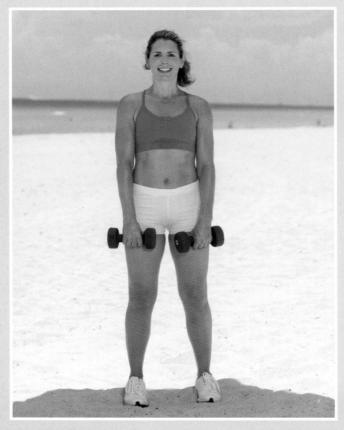

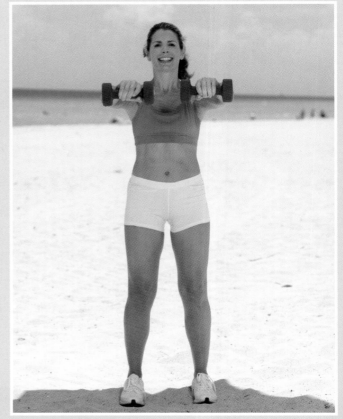

**STARTING POSITION:** Stand with feet hip width apart with soft knees. Hold an 8- to 10-pound (4 to 5 kg) dumbbell in each hand. Straighten your arms so the dumbbells touch the tops of your thighs, knuckles face up.

**TIPS AND TRICKS**

- Don't lift your shoulders to your ears; use your shoulder muscles to lift the arms, not your delicate shoulder joints.
- Don't swing your arms; momentum is a no-no when lifting your dumbbells.

**POSITION 1:** Lift the dumbbells straight in front of you. Pause slightly, and then return to the starting position. Do 15 to 20 reps.

## THE PAYOFF:

Develops killer shoulders.

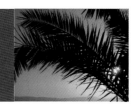

# WEDNESDAY: BURNING FAT WITH CARDIO INTERVALS

On Wednesday, repeat Monday's cardio interval workout, p. 21.

# THURSDAY: GETTING ANOTHER ALL OVER MAKEOVER

On Thursday, repeat Tuesday's allover makeover, p. 22.

# FRIDAY: BURNING FAT WITH CARDIO INTERVALS

On Friday, repeat Monday's cardio interval workout, p. 21.

# SATURDAY: ACHIEVING LOVELY ABS WITH PILATES

If you want the sexiest, most feminine, yet fittest abs ever, do Pilates! I've seen bulky women slim down all over with Pilates. So, let's kick off your Pilates bikini body with abs. This routine is the foundation of the exercises, and you'll be adding other exercises and intensity levels as the weeks go on. Do the exercises in order as Joseph Pilates designed them to streamline your muscles symmetrically. Follow all directions, including the breathing patterns. Don't forget to run through your mental and verbal checklist: head, neck, shoulders, and hips (see the introduction for more Pilates tips, including how to start in the Pilates "V"). The exercises increase in difficulty, so keep reminding yourself to stay within proper alignment and engage your mind. And remember to scoop your abs to your spine the whole time—no bulgy belly!

The following are the Pilates exercises you'll be doing today:

- The Hundred
- Roll-up
- Single Leg Circle
- Rolling Like a Ball
- Single Leg Stretch
- Double Leg Stretch
- Spine Stretch
- Corkscrew
- Saw
- Swan
- Child's Pose
- Single Leg Kick
- Shoulder Bridge
- Teaser 1
- The Seal

# The Hundred

REPLAY WEEKS TWO, THREE, FOUR, FIVE, SIX

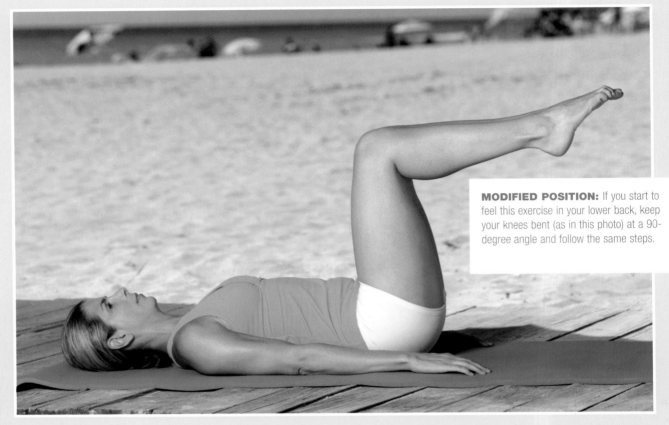

**MODIFIED POSITION:** If you start to feel this exercise in your lower back, keep your knees bent (as in this photo) at a 90-degree angle and follow the same steps.

**STARTING POSITION:** Lie on your back with your knees bent, feet hip width apart. Lengthen your arms by your sides, palms down.

### TIPS AND TRICKS

- Don't bounce your torso as your arms move up and down; focus on your exhale to engage your abs, belly button to spine.
- Don't gasp for breath; keep it flowing from inhale to exhale; it's okay if you can't make it to a count of 5, do what you can.

- Don't tense your neck or clench your jaw; relax, neck tension is so not sexy! If you feel any strain, put a hand behind your head for support. Remember, strong abs can help lift your head. When they're weak, you may feel tension in your neck. Do what you can, but always protect your neck. Rest if you need it!
- Don't let your lower back come off the mat; melt your spine to the mat, using your abs to protect your lower back.

## THE PAYOFF:

Leads to sexy, strong abs and a killer figure.

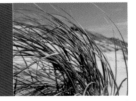

**POSITION 1:** In one motion, straighten your legs to the ceiling, feet in the Pilates "V." Curl your chin to your chest to lift your shoulders off the floor, keep your neck long. Lift and lengthen your arms past your hips, palms down, and begin pumping your arms by your sides.

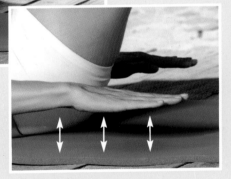

**POSITION 2:** Keeping your wrists straight, inhale to stretch your fingertips long, and pump your arms about 6 to 8 inches (15 to 20 cm) off the floor, as if you're moving your arms through thick molasses, for a count of 5, and then exhale for 5 breaths, emptying your lungs completely to drop your abs to your spine. This completes one breath cycle. Complete 10 breath cycles, thus adding up to The Hundred.

# Roll-up

REPLAY WEEKS TWO, THREE, FOUR

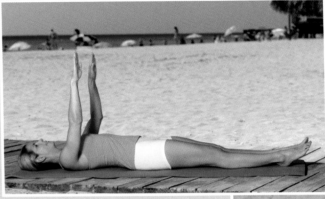

**STARTING POSITION:** Lie on your back with your legs straight, feet in Pilates "V." Straighten your arms so your fingertips reach to the ceiling. Drop the backs of your shoulders against the mat, and slide your shoulder blades down your back.

**TIPS AND TRICKS**

- Don't lift your shoulders to your ears; instead, drop your armpits to your hips.

- Don't jerk up; if you can't roll up in a controlled motion, bend your knees and grab the backs of your thighs to help you.

- Don't plop down; control is crucial, so try rolling down as you press your heels away from your hips. Stay heavy in your heinie!

- Don't forget to squeeze your inner thighs. Place a rolled-up hand towel between your legs to work your inner thighs.

- Don't crane your neck; look at your belly to keep your head in line with your spine the whole time.

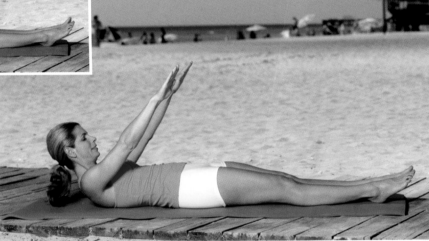

**POSITION 1:** Inhale to curl your chin to your chest, lifting the backs of your shoulders off the mat to look between your arms, keep your neck long. Peel your spine off the mat as if it were a string of pearls.

**THE PAYOFF:**

Develops strong, flat abs and a flexible, healthy spine.

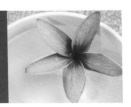

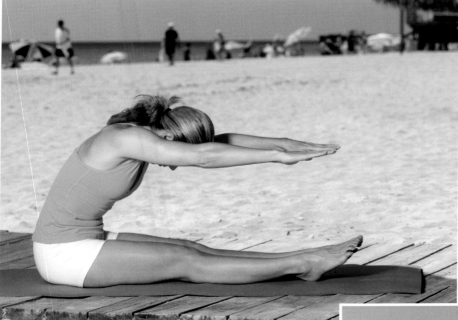

**POSITION 2:** Exhale to round over, scooping your abs to your spine. Reach your fingers past your toes and flex your feet to stretch your hamstrings.

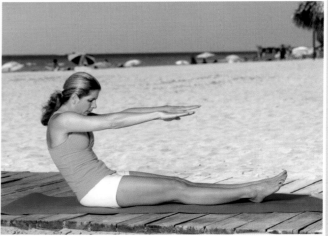

**POSITION 3:** Inhale to lift your pubic bone toward the ceiling, and exhale to roll down, vertebra by vertebra, to the start position. Repeat 3 to 5 times. Don't forget to scoop your abs.

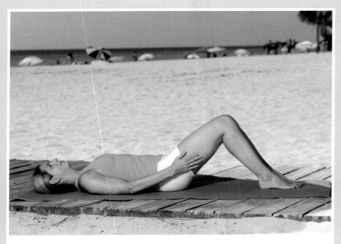

**MODIFIED POSITION:** If you're a beginner or feel any strain in your lower back, you can also start with your knees bent.

# Single Leg Circle

REPLAY WEEKS TWO, THREE, FOUR, FIVE, SIX

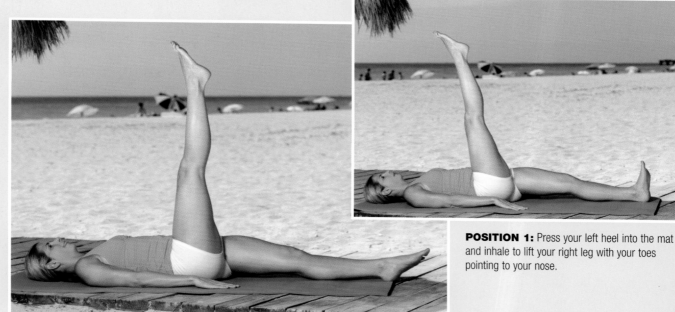

**POSITION 1:** Press your left heel into the mat and inhale to lift your right leg with your toes pointing to your nose.

**STARTING POSITION:** Lie on your back with your left leg straight on the floor while your right leg is at a 90-degree angle, toes reaching long to the ceiling. Straighten your arms by your sides, palms down. Drop the backs of your shoulders against the mat, and slide your shoulder blades down your back.

## TIPS AND TRICKS

- Don't rock your hips from side to side as the leg circles; fire up your core and keep your circles small at first.
- Press the palms of your hands, the backs of your arms, and the back of your head firmly into the mat, which will help stabilize you.
- Don't forget to exhale deeply to stabilize your torso and strengthen your abs.

# THE PAYOFF:

Develops sexy, flat abs and takes inches off your thighs.

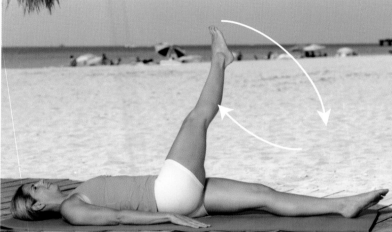

**POSITION 2:** Exhale to move the right leg across your body, inner thighs active.

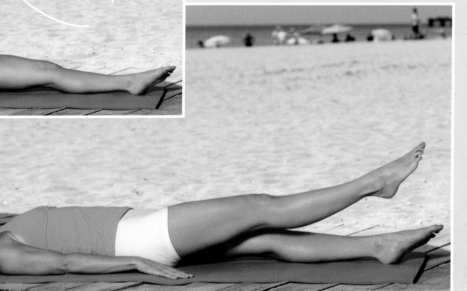

**POSITION 3:** Continue to exhale while moving your right leg to the opposite foot.

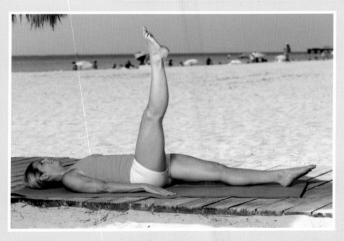

**POSITION 4:** Continue to exhale and circle your leg so it ends up at your nose. Inhale and pause slightly before circling your leg again. Imagine a string pulling your big toe to the ceiling to lengthen your leg as you circle it. Repeat 5 leg circles, and then reverse the circle for 5. Repeat with the left leg.

# Rolling Like a Ball

REPLAY WEEKS TWO, THREE, FOUR, FIVE, SIX

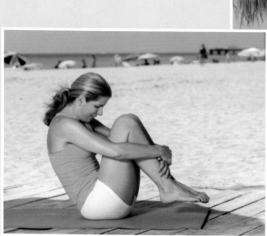

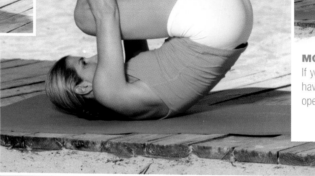

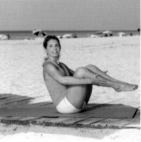

**STARTING POSITION:** Sit at the edge of the mat and slide your booty to your heels. Wrap your arms around your legs, elbows out to the sides. Place your hands on your shins, and cross them at the wrists. Your heels stay close to your bottom. Lower your head between your knees so your spine is rounded, belly button to your spine. Lift your toes off the floor, about 2 inches (5 cm). Use your belly muscles to balance.

**TIPS AND TRICKS**

- Don't roll on your neck; it's about lifting your fanny to the ceiling and keeping active in your belly so you roll only on your upper back.
- Don't lift your shoulders; instead, drop your armpits to your hips.

**MODIFIED POSITION:** If you're a beginner or are having trouble rolling up, open your knees.

**POSITION 1:** Inhale to roll back to the middle portion of your back, scooping your abs and lifting your booty to the ceiling. Stay rounded so that you don't roll back onto your head. Exhale to lift through your pelvic floor and scoop your abs for extra power to roll up and balance. Imagine you're a ball in motion. Repeat 8 to 10 times.

## THE PAYOFF:

Leads to a healthy, strong, and flexible spine.

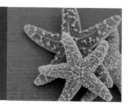

# Single Leg Stretch

REPLAY WEEKS THREE, FOUR

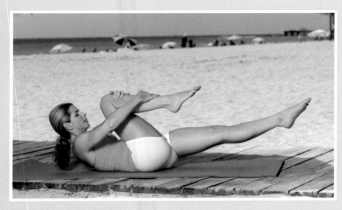

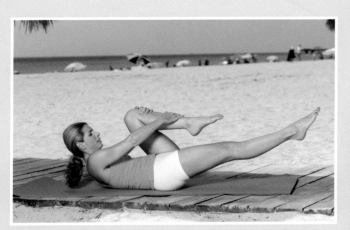

**STARTING POSITION:** Lie on your back with your knees to your chest. Place your right hand on the outside of your right shin and your left hand just below your knee, elbows out to your sides. In one motion, inhale to curl your chin to your chest to lift your shoulders off the ground and straighten your left leg so your toes are in line with your nose while giving your right knee two little hugs.

**TIPS AND TRICKS**

- Don't freak out about the hand placement; it keeps your knee in line with your ankle and hip, but if you get totally frustrated, just clasp your hands and place them behind your head for support.

- Don't rock from side to side while moving your legs; engage your abs to stay stable in your torso.

- Don't bend your knees; as you move your legs away from your torso, stretch them as far as possible.

- Don't look at the ceiling; look between your thighs to maintain proper head placement and work those abs.

- Single Leg Stretch is part of the best ab strengthening and toning series called "The Fives." A second one in the series, Double Leg Stretch, follows this exercise; the other three are presented in Week Three. Keep going, Double Leg Stretch is next.

**POSITION 1:** Continue to inhale and switch legs, bringing your left knee to your chest while your left hand is on your left shin and your right hand is just below your knee, give your knee two hugs. Exhale to switch legs to bring your right knee to your chest, right hand on right shin and left hand on the knee; continue exhaling to switch legs to bring your left knee to your chest, left hand on shin and right hand on knee; this is one set. Exhale gradually to flatten your belly. Repeat 5 to 10 times.

# THE PAYOFF:

Gives you flat, sexy, strong abs.

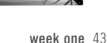

# Double Leg Stretch

REPLAY WEEKS TWO, THREE, FOUR

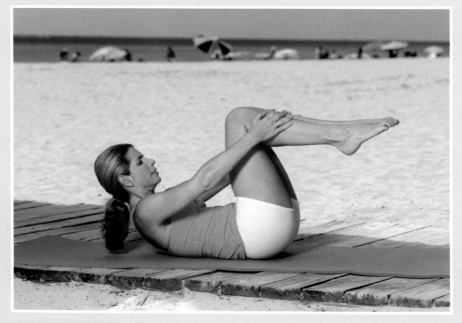

**STARTING POSITION:** Lie on your back with your knees to your chest and place your hands on your shins. Curl your chin to your chest and lift your head, neck, and upper back off the mat.

**TIPS AND TRICKS**

- Don't look at the ceiling; keep your chin to your chest and look between your thighs at all times. If you still feel tension, your abs might not be strong enough yet. Rest your head off the mat and move it from side to side between the two exercises.

- Don't bounce, jerk, or lift your lower back from the mat while your arms and legs move; your arms and legs are challenging your abs, so use them by scooping your belly button to your spine the whole time.

- Don't arch your back as your legs move away from your torso; keep your back flat against the mat the whole time. If you can't maintain a flat back, straighten your legs to the ceiling to reduce the stress on your lower back.

## THE PAYOFF:

Develops crazy-strong, flat abs.

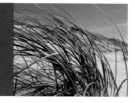

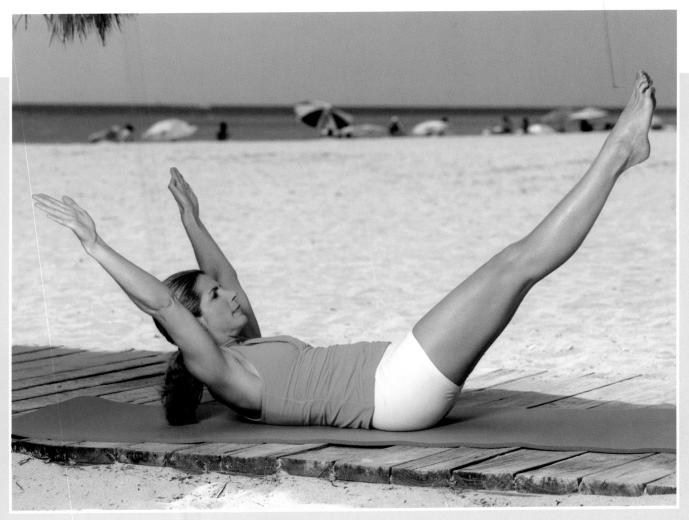

**POSITION 1:** In one motion, inhale to straighten your legs to the ceiling and reach your arms over your head, and begin to circle them behind you and around. Exhale to finish the circle, then use your abs to bring your knees to your chest. Give your knees a hug with your hands to empty your lungs of air—it's a lovely lower back stretch. Repeat 5 to 8 smooth flowing stretches.

# Spine Stretch

REPLAY WEEKS TWO, THREE, FOUR, FIVE, SIX

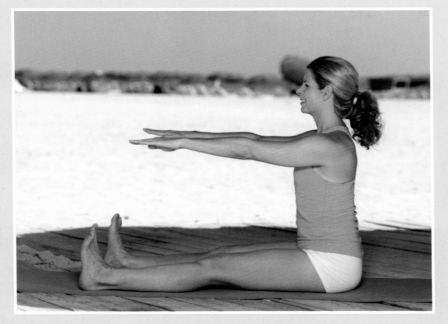

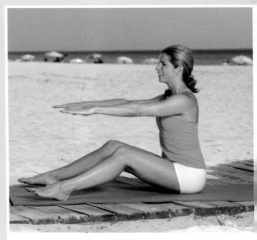

**STARTING POSITION:** Sit on your mat with your legs straight, a little wider than shoulder width apart, feet flexed. Practice perfect posture (shoulders over hips; shoulder blades sliding down your back; sitting on top of your butt bones; head lengthening to the ceiling). Lift your arms so they're parallel to your legs. Inhale to grow tall in your spine.

### TIPS AND TRICKS

- Don't move your lower body; turn on your hamstrings and flex your feet as you round over.
- Don't stretch forward; scoop your abs to stretch your spine and round over. You may feel a lovely hamstrings stretch, too.
- Don't slump in your lower back; sit on top of your butt bones, as though you're sitting on hot rocks.

**MODIFIED POSITION:** If you have tight hamstrings and you're slumping in your lower back, modify the position by bending your knees or putting a small pad under your bottom.

## THE PAYOFF:

Develops a healthy, flexible spine.

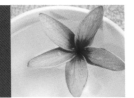

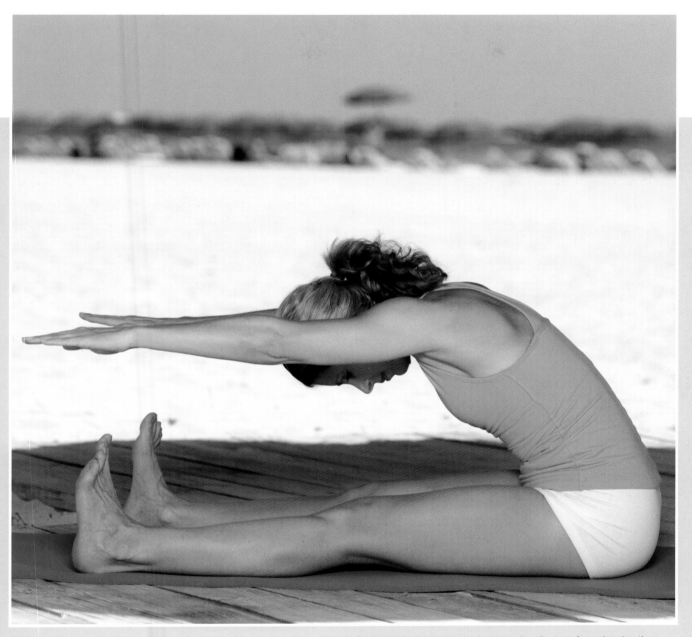

**POSITION 1:** Exhale to round over, curling the top of your head to the floor; imagine a mean, ugly porcupine with long sharp, needles under your belly—scoop, scoop, scoop! As your fingertips stretch past your toes, scoop your abs to feel the stretch in your lower back. Inhale to roll up, vertebra on top of vertebra. Repeat 3 to 5 times.

# Corkscrew

REPLAY WEEKS TWO, THREE, FOUR, FIVE, SIX

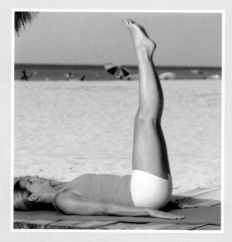

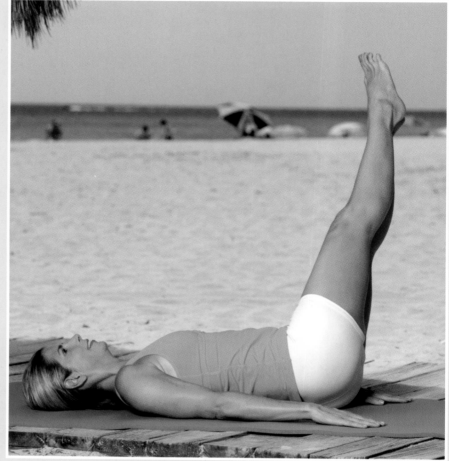

**STARTING POSITION:** Lie on your back with your legs straight at a 90-degree angle, feet in a Pilates "V." Straighten your arms by your sides, pressing the palms of your hands into the mat. Slide your shoulder blades down your back.

### TIPS AND TRICKS

- Don't lift your head or shoulders off the mat; keep your circles small so you can maintain good form until you get strong enough.

- Don't separate your legs; squeeze your inner thighs to give you lots of power!

- Don't forget to use the power of your arms by pressing into the mat to lift your hips.

**POSITION 1:** Make a small circle with your legs to the left, letting the right hip come off the mat slightly. Keep your knees and ankles together the entire time.

## THE PAYOFF:

Scorches those love handles.

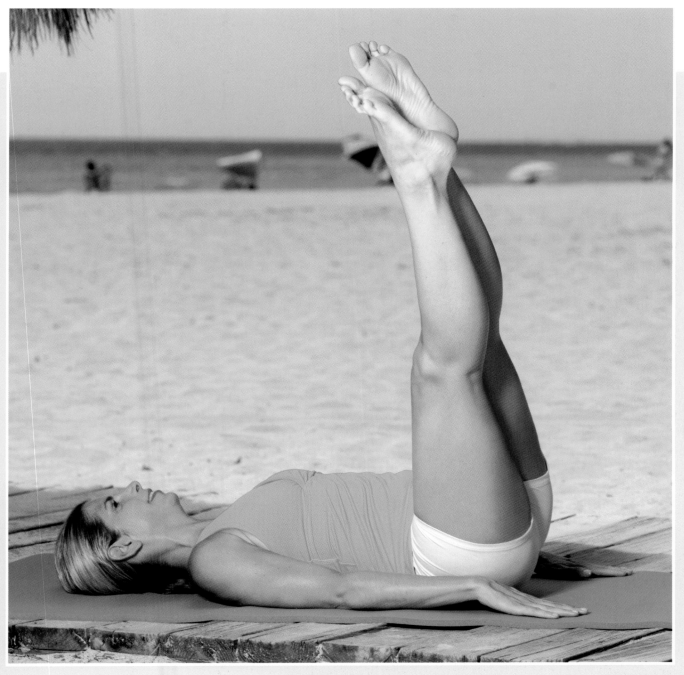

**POSITION 2:** Complete the circle to the right. Reverse the direction, circle left and finish right; that's one complete set. Imagine a string pulling your toes to the ceiling, so lengthen your legs away from your hips, keeping your knees and ankles together. Do 3 to 5 circles.

# Saw

REPLAY WEEKS TWO, THREE, FOUR, FIVE, SIX

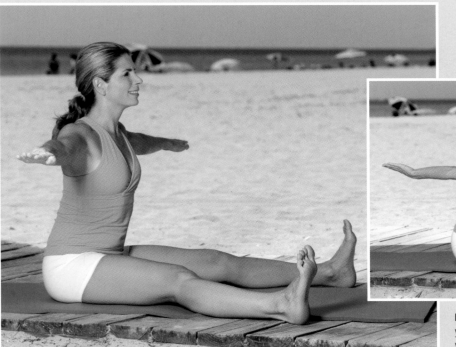

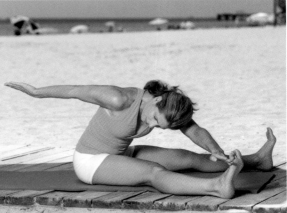

**STARTING POSITION:** Sit tall on the mat with your legs straight and a little wider than shoulder width apart, feet flexed. Lift your arms out to the sides of your body, and reach your fingertips long, palms down. Inhale to grow tall in your spine, lifting your ribs slightly up off your pelvis to initiate the twist.

## TIPS AND TRICKS

- Don't bounce as you twist; it's a lengthening from your waist as you reach your arms farther apart.

- Don't do any rotation if you have a back injury; please ask your doctor if "rotation" or "twisting" is appropriate for you.

- Don't slump in your lower back; sit on top of your butt bones like you're sitting on hot rocks!

**POSITION 1:** Exhale to reach your left hand to your right foot and past the pinky toe—imagine your left pinky finger "sawing" off your right pinky toe while your left ear moves closer to your right knee; pulse for 3 counts while stretching your right hand behind you, palm up. With each pulse, twist a little farther, exhaling every ounce of air from your lungs as if you were wringing out a dirty dish towel. Inhale to return to the starting position even taller in your spine.

# THE PAYOFF:

Leads to a stunning waist and strong obliques.

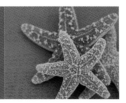

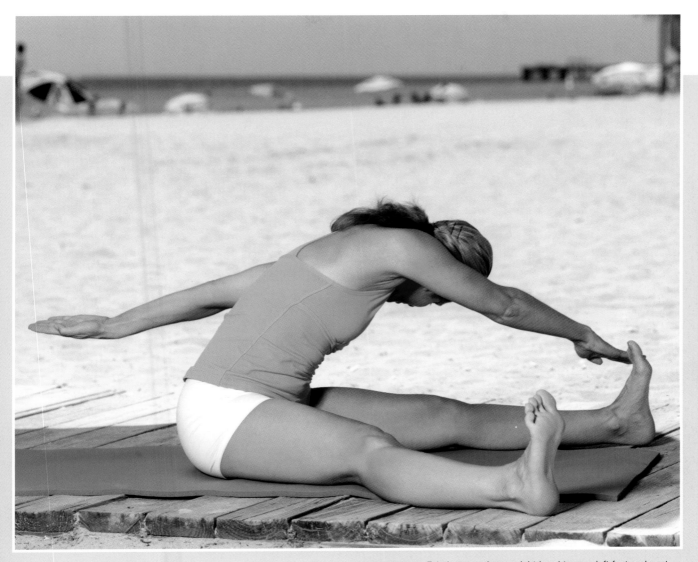

**POSITION 2:** Exhale to reach your right hand to your left foot and past the pinky toe. Imagine sawing off your pinky toe while your right ear moves closer to your left knee; pulse for 3 counts while stretching your left hand behind you, palm up. With each pulse, twist a little farther, exhaling every ounce of air out of your lungs. Inhale to return to the starting position even taller in your spine. Repeat 3 to 5 times.

# Swan

REPLAY WEEKS TWO, THREE, FOUR, FIVE, SIX

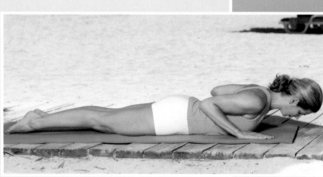

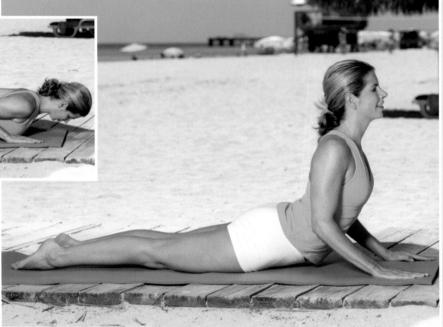

**STARTING POSITION:** Lie on your stomach with your legs straight, placing your hands directly under your shoulders, palms down. Elbows are close to your rib cage. Put some action in your butt cheeks and lift your belly button toward your spine.

### TIPS AND TRICKS

- Don't forget about the principles of extension: hip bones and pubic bone press into the mat; booty and hamstrings are engaged; armpits are dropped to your hips.

- Don't move your elbows to the sides of your chest; imagine a pencil between your arms and your rib cage, then squeeze it and shave your elbows past your rib cage to keep your elbows close to your body.

- Don't elevate your shoulders as you rock up and down; lower your shoulder blades down your back to stabilize your shoulders and open your chest.

**POSITION 1:** Inhale and slowly lift your chest off the mat, leading with your breastbone. Lift as high as you can, without feeling any pressure in your lower back. Exhale, lower to the mat, and quickly inhale up so you're rocking on your belly. Repeat 3 to 5 times.

## THE PAYOFF:

Gives you a healthy belly and strong, fit back.

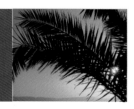

# Child's Pose

REPLAY WEEK TWO

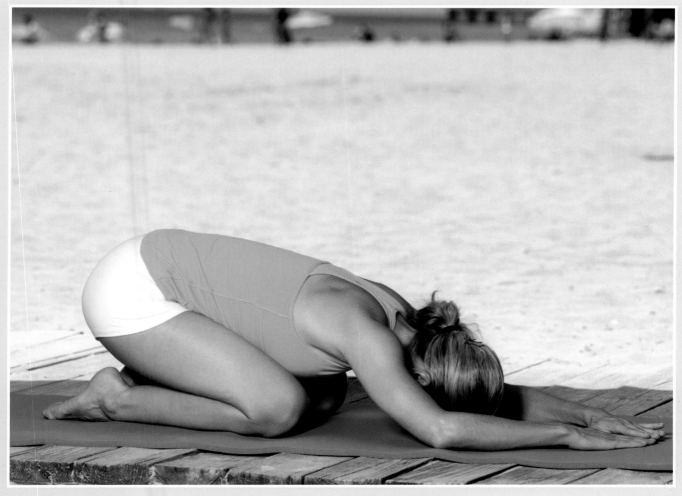

**STARTING POSITION:** Lie on your belly and slide your bum to rest on your heels.

**POSITION 1:** Move your arms over your head and breathe normally.

**TIPS AND TRICKS**

- Don't strain your knees; if you have any pain, put a blanket between your knees and your bum.

## THE PAYOFF:

Makes for an oh-so-yummy stretch for your back.

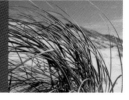

# Single Leg Kick

REPLAY WEEKS TWO, THREE, FOUR, FIVE, SIX

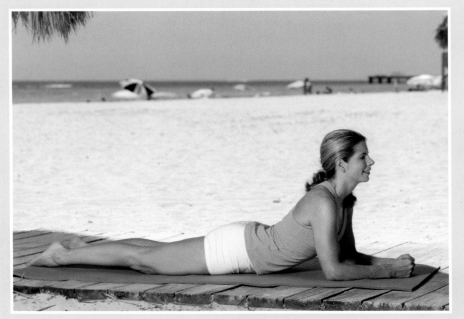

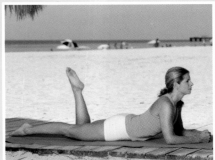

**POSITION 1:** Inhale, kick your right heel to your butt and then kick again.

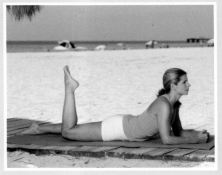

**POSITION 2:** Exhale, kick your right heel to your butt, and then kick again. Keep a steady rhythm going, both legs should be moving at the same time. Repeat 5 to 8 times.

**STARTING POSITION:** Lie on your stomach and lift your belly button toward your spine. Firm up your fanny and press your hip bones and pubic bone into the mat. Put your elbows directly under your shoulders and toward the belly to make an upside down "V," and press your elbows into the mat. Make two fists, and place your knuckles together.

**TIPS AND TRICKS**

- Don't jiggle your booty; keep your pelvis stable and firm up your fanny.
- Don't round your shoulders; lift your head out of your shoulders as your breastbone lifts to the ceiling.
- Don't sag your belly; stay active to support your lower back. If you feel any lower back strain, put a pillow underneath your pelvis.

## THE PAYOFF:

Firms up your backside.

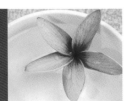

# Shoulder Bridge

REPLAY WEEK TWO

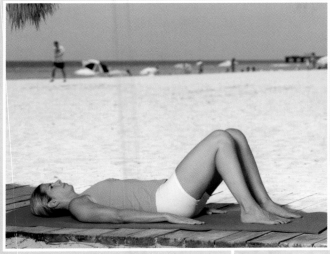

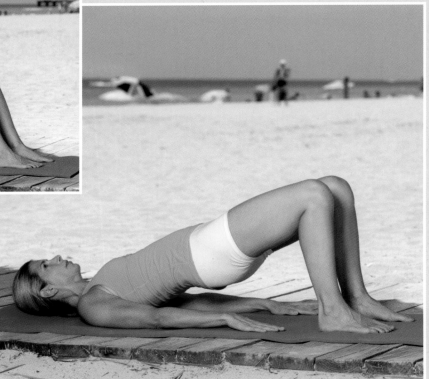

**STARTING POSITION:** Lie on your back with your arms straight by your sides and place your feet about hip width apart. Inhale to cue your body.

**TIPS AND TRICKS**

- Don't sag in your booty; keep your hips even and maintain a neutral position to build your core strength.
- Don't forget to use your abs; stay solid from your breastbone to your pubic bone so you don't sink in your hips.

**POSITION 1:** Exhale to scoop your abs and lift your spine off the mat, vertebra by vertebra, and then inhale to roll down, vertebra by vertebra. Imagine a sling hangs from the ceiling to hoist your hips to prevent your bottom from sinking into the mat. Repeat 3 to 5 times.

## THE PAYOFF:

Develops an incredibly strong core and perks up your booty.

# Teaser 1

REPLAY WEEK TWO

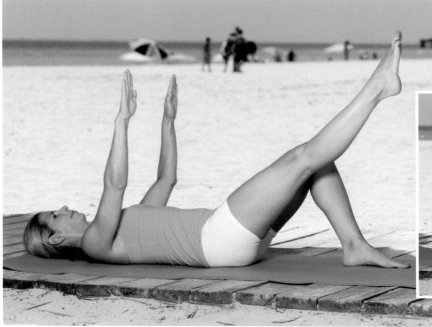

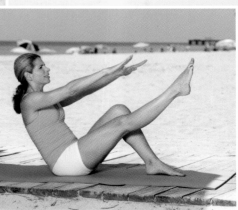

**STARTING POSITION:** Lie on your back with your right leg straight and your left knee bent, foot on the mat, while straightening your arms to the ceiling.

**TIPS AND TRICKS**

- Don't strain in your lower back; use your abs to lift up or hold the backs of your legs if you don't have the belly strength.
- Don't plop down; scoop and uncurl your spine to lower to the mat with control.

**POSITION 1:** At the same time, inhale to lift your arms to your right leg in a "V," fingertips reaching for your toes. Scoop, scoop, scoop to build strength and protect your lower back. Exhale to roll down slowly to the mat. Repeat 3 to 5 times.

## THE PAYOFF:

Gives you oh-so stunning abs.

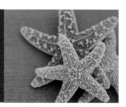

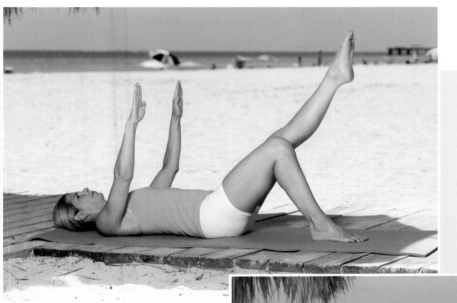

**POSITION 2:** Lie on your back with your left leg straight and your right knee bent, foot on the mat, while straightening your arms to the ceiling.

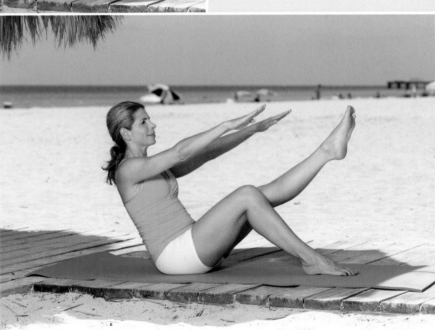

**POSITION 3:** At the same time, inhale to lift your arms to your left leg in a "V," fingertips reaching for your toes. Scoop, scoop, scoop to build strength and protect your lower back. Exhale to roll down slowly to the mat. Repeat 3 to 5 times.

# The Seal

REPLAY WEEKS TWO, THREE, FOUR, FIVE, SIX

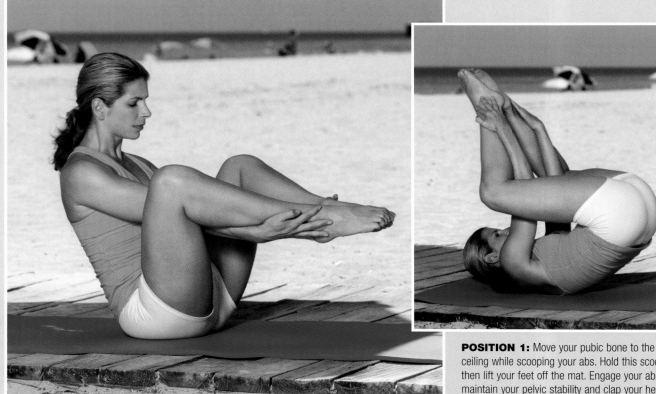

**STARTING POSITION:** Sit at the edge of the mat and slide your heels to your booty. Drive into your legs and wrap your arms under and around so your hands end up on the outside of your ankles. Look at your belly as you drop your chin to your chest, rounding your spine.

**TIPS AND TRICKS**

- Don't forget to engage your inner thighs when you clap your heels.
- Don't roll onto your head or neck; it's the upper back and shoulders that absorb the weight of your body.

**POSITION 1:** Move your pubic bone to the ceiling while scooping your abs. Hold this scoop, then lift your feet off the mat. Engage your abs to maintain your pelvic stability and clap your heels and bark like a seal. (Why not? It's free and fun.) Inhale to roll back to your upper back, only. Exhale to roll up. Pause, clap your heels 3 times, and roll again, scooping your belly the whole time to find your balance. Repeat 8 to 10 times.

## THE PAYOFF:

Leads to a flexible, fit spine.

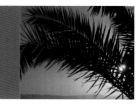

# SUNDAY: PUTTING YOUR (BEAUTIFUL) TOES UP

Take this day off to get some much-needed rest. But let this still be a great bikini day, by adding some healthy eating habits that will get you bikini ready:

- **Drink plenty of water:** Drink eight 8-ounce glasses of water throughout the day, starting first thing in the morning.

- **Eat breakfast:** If you skip breakfast, you usually end up overeating the rest of the day, so fix something small and nutritious. Mix and match sliced apples and almond butter (yummy), toast with almond butter, cereal with mixed berries, or a smoothie.

- **Banish nighttime eating:** The nighttime munchies are oh-so-bad for your bikini body. Eat dinner by 6:00 p.m. and nothing else. The best way to achieve your bikini body is to eat your biggest meal at lunch, and then have a small meal, such as a salad, at 6:00 p.m. (I love having low-fat or 2 percent yogurt for dinner, because then I know I'll have great energy for my bikini workout the next day.)

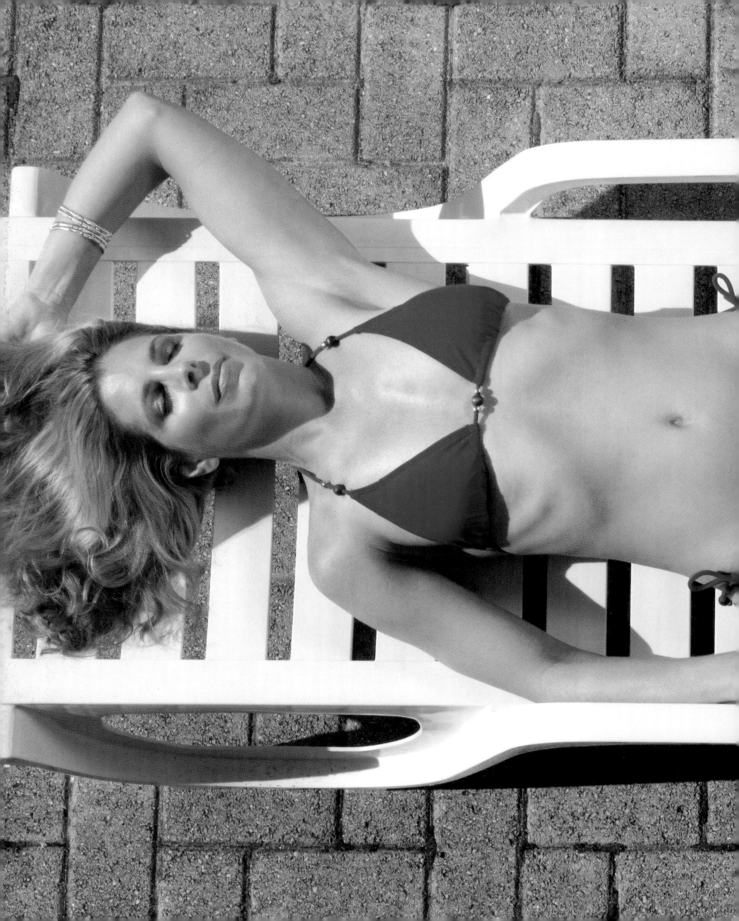

# week two

## NO JUNK IN YOUR TRUNK

To get rid of the junk in your trunk, you have to burn fat. To burn fat, you have to build muscle. This week, you'll move with strength intervals to fight fat even faster. Strength intervals keep your heart rate up so the pounds melt away, all while building sexy muscles. In the end, more muscles burn more calories a day, every day, and you'll have less junk in your bikini trunk.

Keep in mind that mixing weights with an aerobic workout can give you the best combination of all to burn off fat and maintain muscle at the same time. Preserving or increasing muscle will kick your fat burners into overdrive and give you a bikini body.

| | |
|---|---|
| **MONDAY** | Turning On and Toning Up with Body Boot Camp |
| **TUESDAY** | Getting Lean with Cardio |
| **WEDNESDAY** | Using Pilates for a Speedy Butt Lift |
| **THURSDAY** | Turning On and Toning Up with Body Boot Camp |
| **FRIDAY** | Getting Lean with Cardio |
| **SATURDAY** | Using Pilates for a Speedy Butt Lift |
| **SUNDAY** | Letting Go! |

# WORKOUT PROGRAM AT A GLANCE

| MONDAY | TUESDAY | WEDNESDAY | THURSDAY |
|---|---|---|---|
| Turning On and Toning Up with Body Boot Camp | Getting Lean with Cardio | Using Pilates for a Speedy Butt Lift | Turning On and Toning Up with Body Boot Camp |

| MONDAY | TUESDAY | WEDNESDAY | THURSDAY |
|---|---|---|---|
| **Set 1**<br>Walking Lunge<br>Chest Press<br>Triceps Kickbacks | **1.** 3 minutes: Intensity level 4 or 5 to warm up<br><br>**2.** 50 minutes: Intensity level 7 to 9 (heavy breathing and sweaty)<br><br>**3.** 2 minutes: Intensity level 3 or 4 to cool down | **After doing the Pilates Abs in week one, do the following exercises today:**<br>Side Kick Front<br>Beat … Beat … UP<br>Side Passé<br>Single Leg Circle (front and back)<br>Outer Thigh Lift<br>Straight Line Leg Lift<br>Outer Thigh Lift, Close the Hatch, and Pac-Man<br>Scissor Legs<br>Hot Potato<br>Clam<br>Froggy<br>Beat on the Belly | **Set 1**<br>Walking Lunge<br>Chest Press<br>Triceps Kickbacks |
| **Set 2**<br>Plyometric Squat<br>Bent Over Row<br>Biceps Curls | | | **Set 2**<br>Plyometric Squat<br>Bent Over Row<br>Biceps Curls |
| **Set 3**<br>Speedy Steps<br>Reverse Fly<br>Side Arm Raise<br>Front Arm Raise | | | **Set 3**<br>Speedy Steps<br>Reverse Fly<br>Side Arm Raise<br>Front Arm Raise |

| **FRIDAY** | **SATURDAY** | **SUNDAY** |
|---|---|---|
| Getting Lean with Cardio | Using Pilates for a Speedy Butt Lift | Letting Go! |

**FRIDAY — Getting Lean with Cardio**

1. 3 minutes: Intensity level 4 or 5 to warm up
2. 50 minutes: Intensity level 7 to 9 (heavy breathing and sweaty)
3. 2 minutes: Intensity level 3 or 4 to cool down

**SATURDAY — Using Pilates for a Speedy Butt Lift**

**After doing the Pilates Abs in week one, do the following exercises today:**

Side Kick Front

Beat … Beat … UP

Side Passé

Single Leg Circle (front and back)

Outer Thigh Lift

Straight Line Leg Lift

Outer Thigh Lift, Close the Hatch, and Pac-Man

Scissor Legs

Hot Potato

Clam

Froggy

Beat on the Belly

**SUNDAY — Letting Go!**

OFF

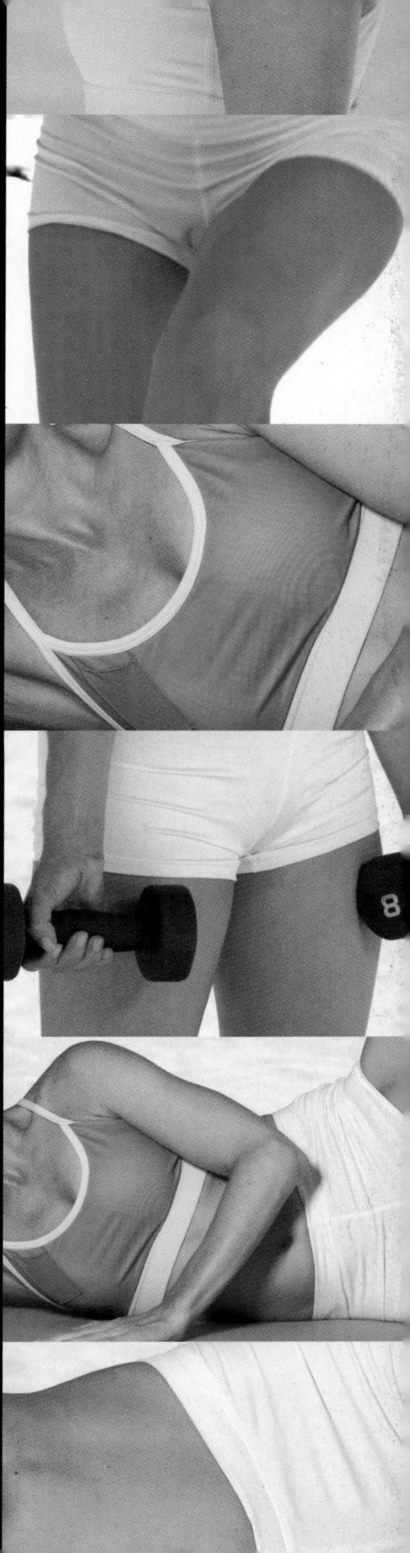

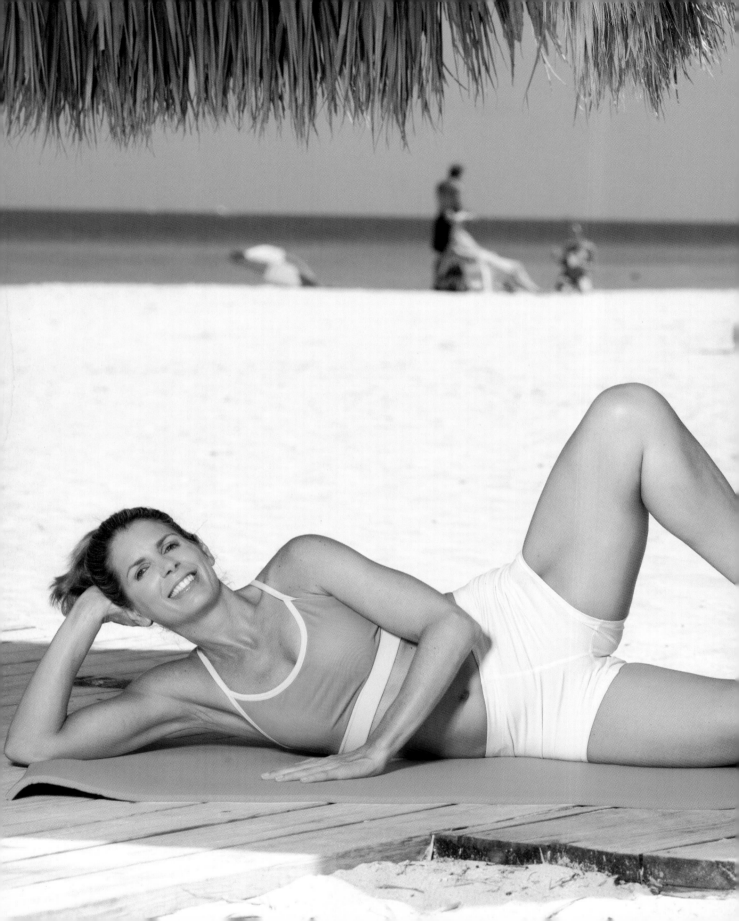

# MONDAY: TURNING ON AND TONING UP WITH BODY BOOT CAMP

Fight fat faster with this high-energy, calorie-burning routine. The exercises on these pages still give you an all over workout, only now you'll turn up the heat for your legs and booty with plyometric moves. To keep things simple, the arm work is the same as in Week one, good news, right? You'll need a couple sets of dumbbells. For your legs and butt, the dumbbells need to be heavy enough to finish a set with good form, which is 15 to 20 pounds (7 to 9 kg) for most women. For your arms, use a lighter pair of dumbbells, 8 to 10 pounds (4 to 5 kg).

To do this boot camp workout you'll do each of the exercises in Set 1 three times, doing 15 to 20 reps of each exercise, and then repeat those three exercises two more times. For example, complete 15 to 20 slow and controlled reps of each of the following exercises: Walking Lunge, Chest Press, and Triceps Kickbacks. Repeat that set two times before moving on to Set 2, and then finish with Set 3. Total time should be about 45 minutes to 1 hour. If you're not clear on what a set or a rep is, flip to the introduction to this book. Also, all boot camp-style routines count as both your cardio and your strength training. So keep your heart rate revving during the entire workout. To do this, you'll move from exercise to exercise with no more than 30 seconds of rest. Your goal is to alternate between low- and high-intensity intervals or, put another way, from a little winded to choppy words (use the intensity scale in the introduction of this book if you need further guidance). Do this workout today and on Thursday. Follow the exercises in order on these pages. And don't forget to warm up on the treadmill for 5 minutes at 3.5 mph (5.5 kph), no grade (which means no incline).

**Set 1**

Walking Lunge

Chest Press

Triceps Kickbacks

**Set 2**

Plyometric Squat

Bent Over Row

Biceps Curls

**Set 3**

Speedy Steps

Reverse Fly

Side Arm Raise

Front Arm Raise

# Walking Lunge

REPLAY WEEK THREE

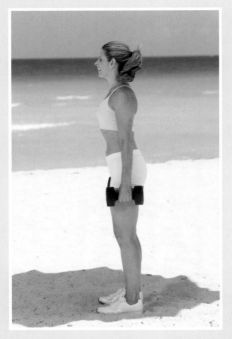

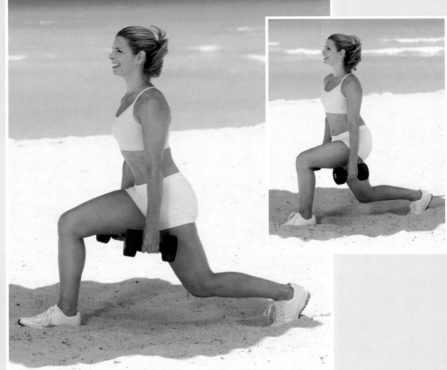

**STARTING POSITION:** Stand with feet hip width apart and hold a 15- to 20-pound (7 to 9 kg) dumbbell in each hand.

Note: You need enough room to walk about 20 steps.

**TIPS AND TRICKS**

- Don't lean forward; align your knee over your second and third toes, keeping your body weight in the lunge leg.

- Don't round your spine; keep your chest lifted, shoulders relaxed, and toes pointing forward.

- Don't forget to use your abs to support your lower back.

**POSITION 1:** Step forward with your right foot to lower your body into a lunge; your right thigh is parallel to the floor while your left thigh is perpendicular to the floor (your left knee should almost touch the floor).

**POSITION 2:** Walk your left foot up to your right foot, come to a standing position, and then lunge forward with the left leg. Keep your spine straight and lifted as you walk. Do 15 to 20 reps.

## THE PAYOFF:

Perks up your butt, gives you strong legs, and blasts fat.

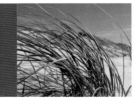

# Chest Press

REPLAY WEEK ONE

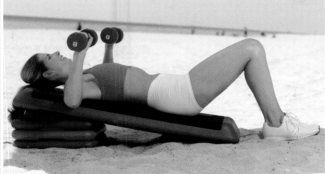

**STARTING POSITION:** Using 8- to 10-pound (4 to 5 kg) dumbbells, lie flat on your back, either on the bench or a step. Lower your arms out to the sides until your elbows are in line with your shoulders so you can see the weights in your peripheral vision. You may feel a slight stretch in the chest area.

### TIPS AND TRICKS

- Don't swing your arms; use control to lift and lower your weights.
- Don't lift your lower back off the bench; engage your abs to support your lower back. If you can't stabilize your torso, drop down in weight; your weights may be too heavy.

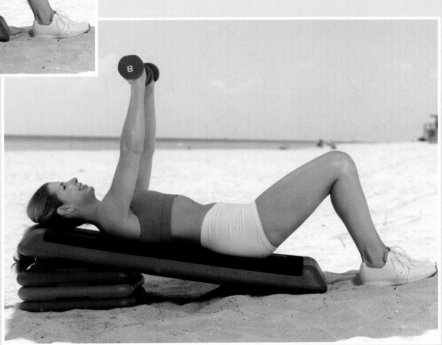

**POSITION 1:** Raise your arms up and together. Pause, and then slowly lower your arms. Do 15 to 20 reps.

## THE PAYOFF:

Develops stunning, sexy, and strong chest.

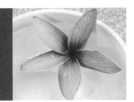

# Triceps Kickbacks

REPLAY WEEK ONE

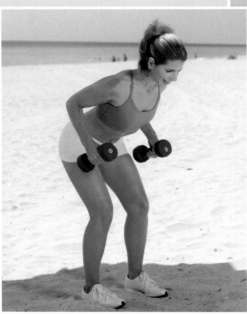

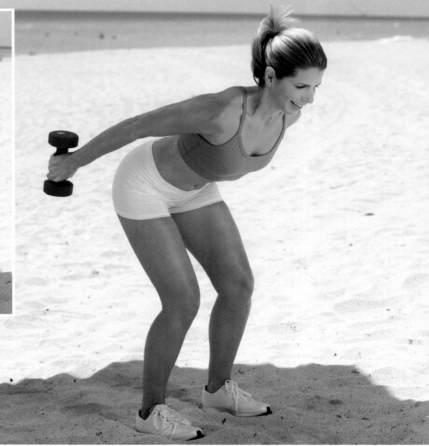

**STARTING POSITION:** Stand in a squat position with an 8- to 10-pound (4 to 5 kg) dumbbell in each hand, knees slightly bent and feet hip width apart. Bend over so that your back is almost parallel to the ground. Bend your elbows to about 90 degrees, raising them to just above your back.

**TIPS AND TRICKS**

- Don't round your spine; keep your abs active and lengthen from the top of your head.

**POSITION 1:** Straighten your arms backward, leading with your pinky finger. Keep your upper arms stationary and near your ribs. When they're fully extended, your arms should be parallel to the ground. Do 15 to 20 reps.

## THE PAYOFF:

Eliminates flabby arms.

I know you're just starting out, but trust me—take care of your body and it will change for the oh-so bikini better. If you find that you need a little inspiration, incentives work! Treat yourself to that mani-pedi, massage, or sexy stilettos when you accomplish your weekly goals—and you'll be on your way to a smoking hot bikini body!

# Plyometric Squat

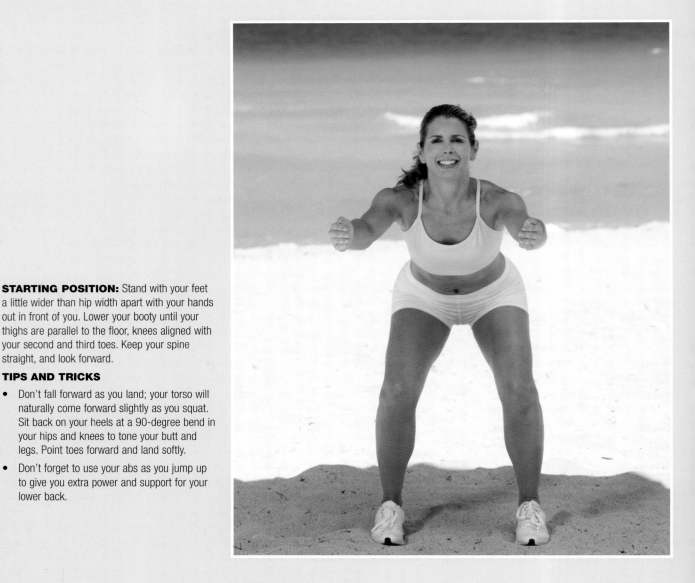

**STARTING POSITION:** Stand with your feet a little wider than hip width apart with your hands out in front of you. Lower your booty until your thighs are parallel to the floor, knees aligned with your second and third toes. Keep your spine straight, and look forward.

**TIPS AND TRICKS**

- Don't fall forward as you land; your torso will naturally come forward slightly as you squat. Sit back on your heels at a 90-degree bend in your hips and knees to tone your butt and legs. Point toes forward and land softly.

- Don't forget to use your abs as you jump up to give you extra power and support for your lower back.

## THE PAYOFF:

Lifts the butt, strengthen the legs, and melts fat.

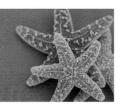

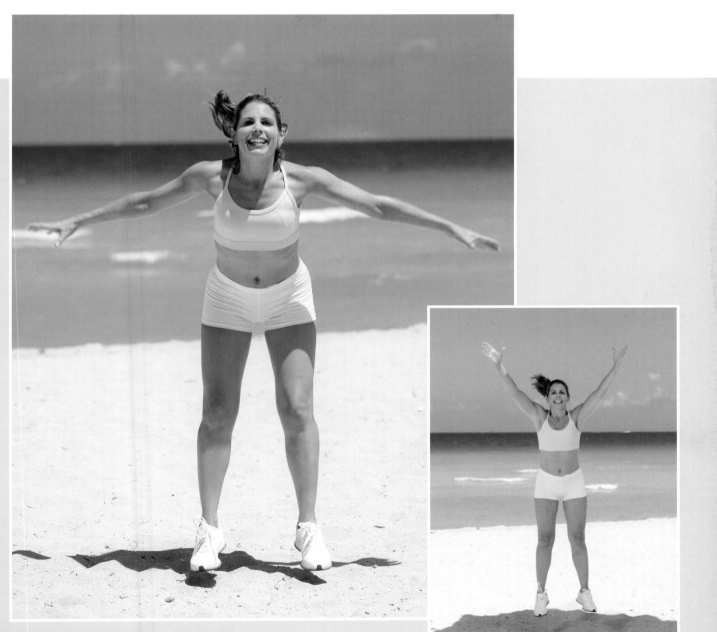

**POSITION 1:** Do three little squat pulses, keeping your booty back as if you were sitting in a chair.

**POSITION 2:** On the fourth rep, jump (think exploding) upward as high as you can, keeping your chest lifted and your spine straight. You can use your arms to help lift you off the ground. Land in a squat and repeat 15 to 20 reps.

# Bent Over Row

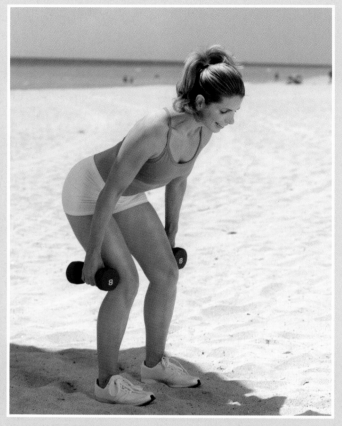

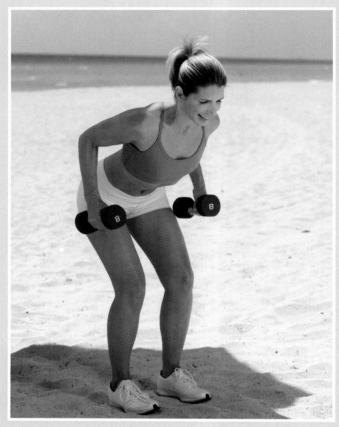

**STARTING POSITION:** Stand with your knees slightly bent and hip width apart. Hold an 8- to 10-pound (4 to 5 kg) dumbbell in each hand and bend from the waist so that your back is almost parallel to the floor. Straighten your arms to the floor, palms facing in.

**TIPS AND TRICKS**
- Don't swing your arms; move with control as your knuckles face out, and keep your elbows in line with your shoulders.

**POSITION 1:** Bend your elbows to lift your dumbbells to the ceiling. The dumbbells will slide on the outside of your chest. Pause and return to the starting position. Do 15 to 20 reps.

## THE PAYOFF:

Sculpts a stunning upper back and strong shoulders.

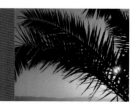

# Biceps Curls

REPLAY WEEK ONE

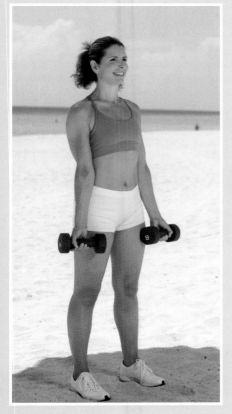

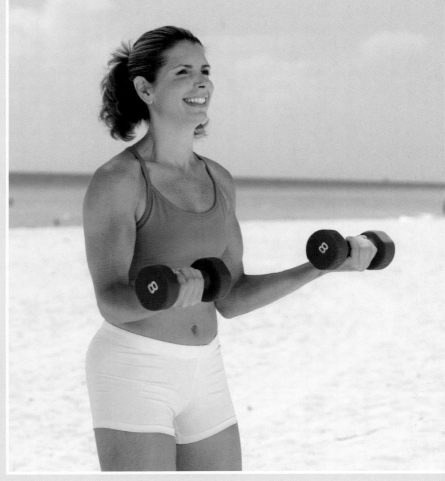

**STARTING POSITION:** Stand with feet hip width apart and hold an 8- to 10-pound (4 to 5 kg) dumbbell in each hand, palms facing up. Straighten your arms so the dumbbells rest just outside of your thighs.

**TIPS AND TRICKS**

- Don't swing your arms as you curl the weight toward your chest.

**POSITION 1:** Keep your elbows close to your torso and curl the dumbbells toward your chest. Do 15 to 20 reps.

## THE PAYOFF:

Overhauls your butt, legs, and core.

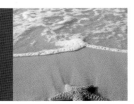

# Speedy Steps

**STARTING POSITION:** Stand about 6 to 12 inches (15 to 30 cm) away from the step or stairs and put the ball of your right foot on the step. Straighten your arms by your sides.

**TIPS AND TRICKS**

- Don't lean forward; keep your torso straight and your head in line with your spine.
- Don't forget to use your abs for extra power.

**POSITION 1:** Quickly switch feet, powering from your legs, not your hips, and keep it going. Do 15 to 20 reps.

## THE PAYOFF:

Gives you a dazzling backside and scorches fat.

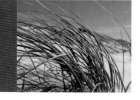

# Reverse Fly

REPLAY WEEK ONE

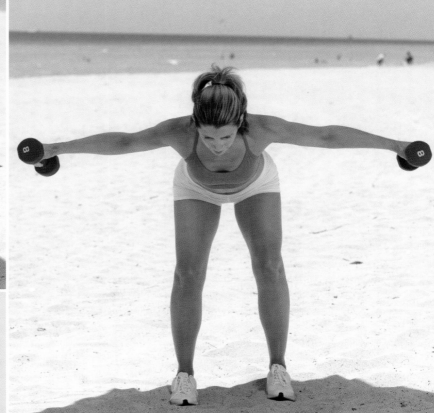

**STARTING POSITION:** Stand with feet hip width apart and in a squat position. Hold an 8- to 10-pound (4 to 5 kg) dumbbell in each hand and bend over from the waist. Turn on your abs to support your lower back. Hang your arms in front, knuckles out, in line with your shoulders.

**TIPS AND TRICKS**

- Don't round your shoulders forward; keep your chest lifted and your shoulders back.
- Don't lift your arms higher than your shoulders; engage your upper back muscles to crack a walnut between your shoulder blades—well, at least imagine it!
- Don't swing your arms; move with control.

**POSITION 1:** Lift your arms up and out to the sides of your body until shoulder height, bringing your shoulder blades together. Your elbows are slightly bent. Do 15 to 20 reps.

## THE PAYOFF:

Gives you a super sexy upper back and strong shoulders.

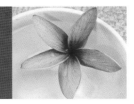

# Side Arm Raise

REPLAY WEEK ONE

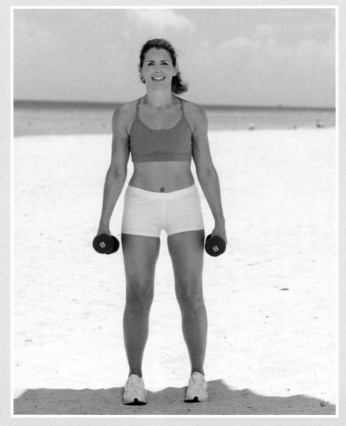 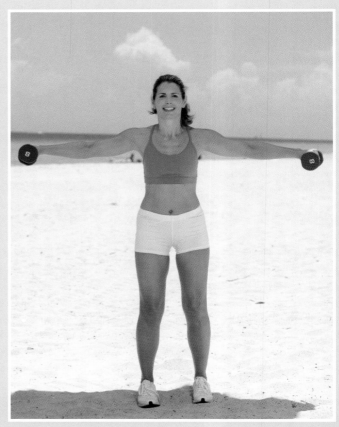

**STARTING POSITION:** Stand with feet hip width apart with soft knees. Hold an 8- to 10-pound (4 to 5 kg) dumbbell in each hand, knuckles face up. Straighten your arms so the dumbbells touch the sides of your thighs, thumbs point in.

**TIPS AND TRICKS**

- Don't bend your wrists; maintain strong arms.
- Don't lift your shoulders to your ears; use your shoulder muscles to lift the arms, not your delicate shoulder joints.

**POSITION 1:** Lift your arms straight out to the sides so the dumbbells end up just below your shoulders. Pause, then return to the starting position. Do 15 to 20 reps.

## THE PAYOFF:

Sculpts strong shoulders.

# Front Arm Raise

REPLAY WEEK ONE

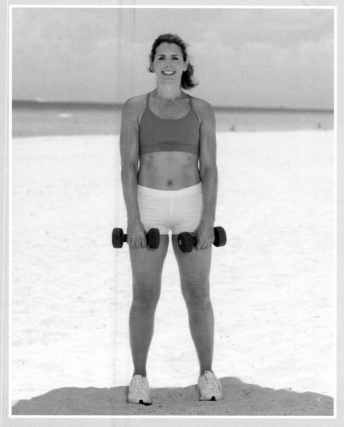

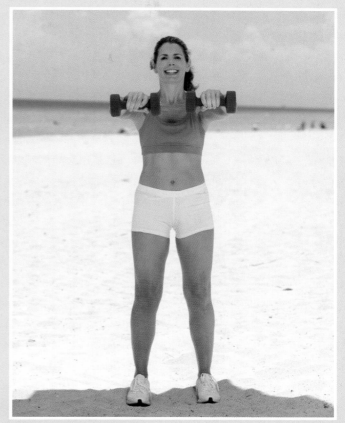

**STARTING POSITION:** Stand with feet hip width apart with soft knees. Hold an 8- to 10-pound (4 to 5 kg) dumbbell in each hand. Straighten your arms so the dumbbells touch the tops of your thighs, knuckles face up.

**POSITION 1:** Lift the dumbbells straight in front of you. Pause slightly, and then return to the starting position. Do 15 to 20 reps.

### TIPS AND TRICKS

- Don't lift your shoulders to your ears; use your shoulder muscles to lift the arms, not your delicate shoulder joints.
- Don't swing your arms; momentum is a no-no when lifting your dumbbells.

## THE PAYOFF:

Develops killer shoulders.

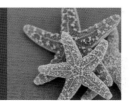

# TUESDAY: GETTING LEAN WITH CARDIO

To keep you from getting injured and your muscles bored, mix up your cardio machines. Today, do a 50- to 55-minute cardio session on an elliptical machine. Warm up for 3 minutes at a level 4 or 5 on the intensity scale (see the introduction of this book for details), and then pick up your speed to a level 7 to 9 (breathing should be heavy and it should be difficult to carry on a full conversation). Push and pull harder so your arms are working as much as your legs. Do this workout today and Friday. Remember, your boot camp workout also counts as your cardio, so this week you'll get four cardio sessions.

If you don't have an elliptical machine at your disposal, see the intensity scale in the introduction of this book to help you determine a similar workout intensity on a treadmill, stair stepper, stationary bike, or by walking or running outside. In the end, it doesn't matter what you do, but how you do it. So sweat it out, keep it physically demanding, but don't over do it.

The following is your workout:

1. 3 minutes: Intensity level 4 or 5 to warm up
2. 50 minutes: Intensity level 7 to 9 (heavy breathing and sweaty)
3. 2 minutes: Intensity level 3 or 4 to cool down

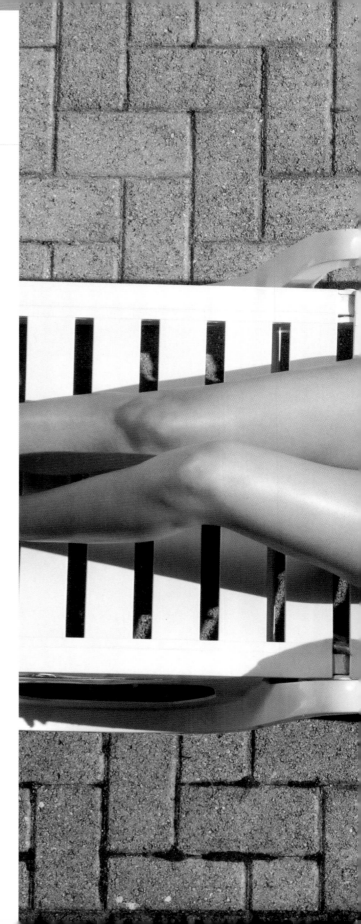

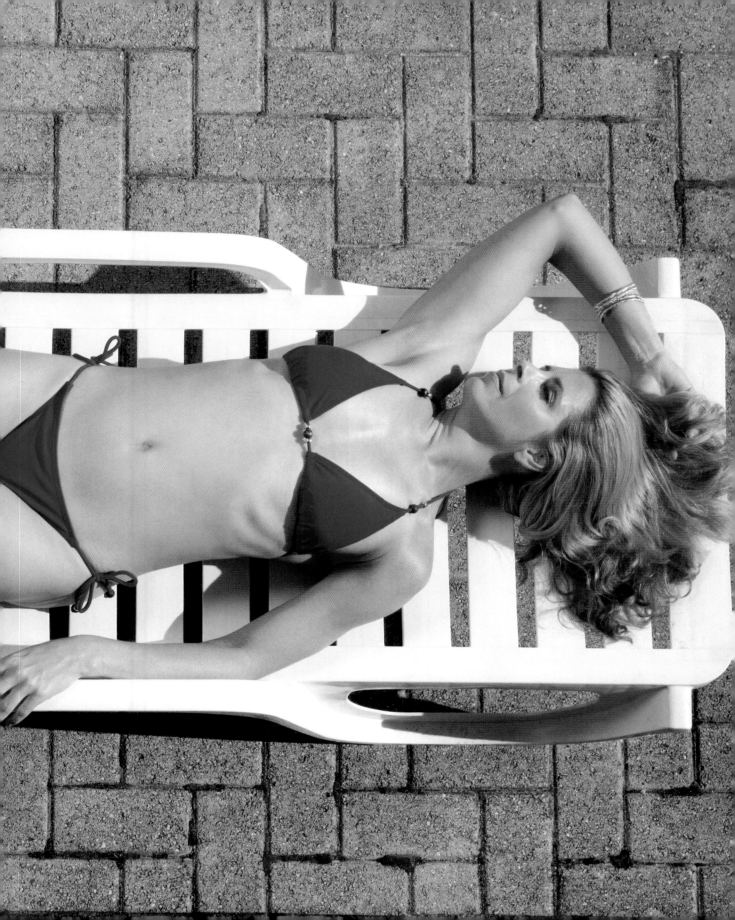

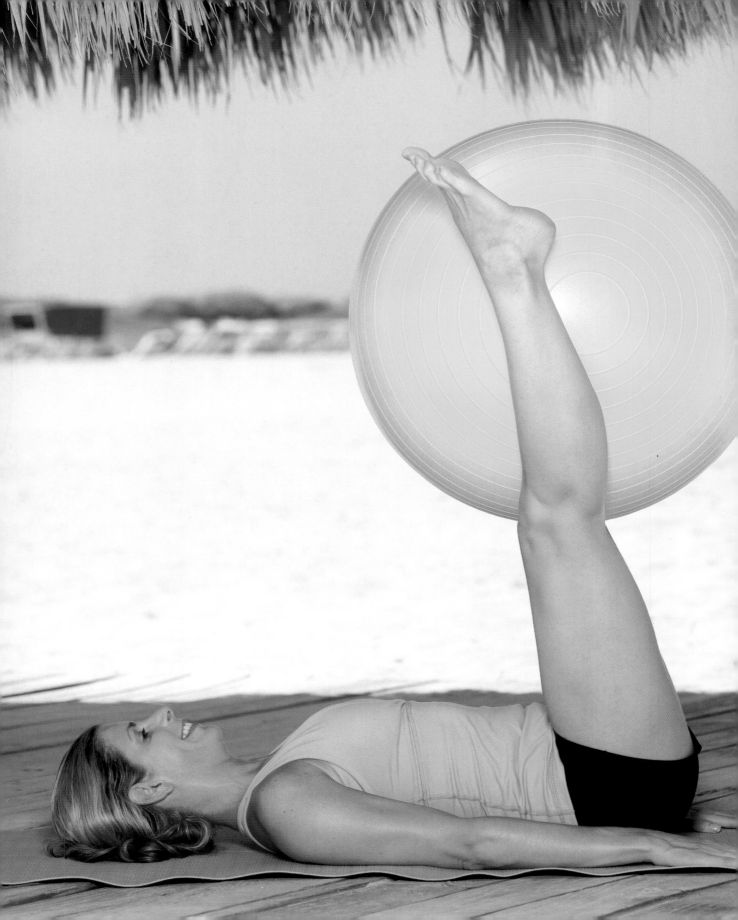

# WEDNESDAY: USING PILATES FOR A SPEEDY BUTT LIFT

The sexiest part of your body is the curve of your hips. So it's time to work your derrière and thighs the Pilates way. This week, do two Pilates sessions with the moves from week one and add the leg exercises from these pages. After doing The Seal from week one, move right into The oh-so-fabulous Side Kick Series. Follow all directions, including the breathing patterns, and shoot for 10 to 20 reps of all exercises unless I state otherwise. Do them in the order shown, left leg first, and then switch sides to do these exact same exercises on the right leg. Don't forget to run through your mental and verbal checklist: head, neck, shoulders, and hips (see the introduction of this book for details).

Note the following starting position for all leg work in this section: lie on your right side with your legs straight; ankles, knees, and hip bones stacked on top of one another; feet in a Pilates "V." Prop your head up with your right arm and then place your left arm, palm down, on the mat in front of your torso; relax your shoulders. Lift both legs at the same time and lower them in front of your body to about a 45-degree angle so your body makes the shape of a banana.

## Pilates Side Kick Series

The Pilates Side Kick Series, which includes the following exercises plus a few of my own favorite leg and butt toners, is fabulous because every exercise tones your trouble zones: legs, butt, and abs. Plus, there's a belly bonus: because your core muscles stabilize you in every exercise, you get extra work for your belly.

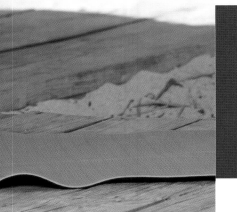

# Side Kick Front

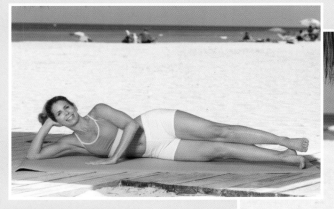

**STARTING POSITION:** Lie on your right side with your legs straight; your ankles, knees, and hip bones stacked on top of one another; and your feet in a Pilates "V." Prop your head up with your right arm and then place your left arm, palm down, on the mat in front of your torso; relax your shoulders. Lift both legs at the same time and lower them in front of your body to about a 45-degree angle so your body makes the shape of a banana.

### TIPS AND TRICKS

- Don't rock and roll in your torso as your leg swings forward and back; use your core muscles to keep you stable and get extra booty work.

**POSITION 1:** Lift your top leg to hip height so it's parallel to the floor, and inhale to swing your leg forward with a kick. Quickly add a smaller kick right after the big kick.

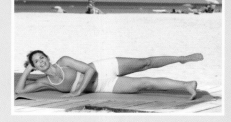

**POSITION 2:** Exhale to swing your leg back and quickly add a small kick to the back to engage your booty.

## THE PAYOFF:

Leads to sexy, strong legs and takes inches off your bottom line.

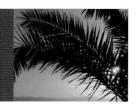

# Beat ... Beat ... UP

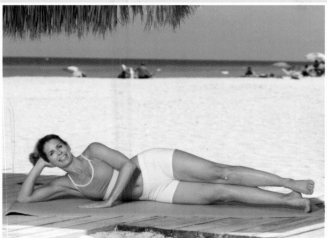

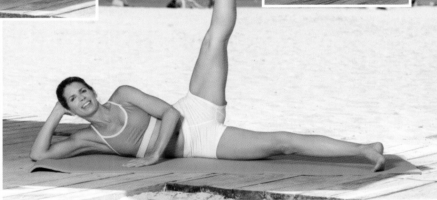

**POSITION 2:** Then exhale to lower the top leg to the bottom, stretching your toes long. Engage your inner thighs to click or beat the top heel to the bottom heel, twice.

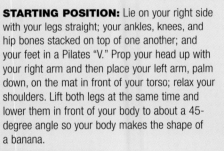

**STARTING POSITION:** Lie on your right side with your legs straight; your ankles, knees, and hip bones stacked on top of one another; and your feet in a Pilates "V." Prop your head up with your right arm and then place your left arm, palm down, on the mat in front of your torso; relax your shoulders. Lift both legs at the same time and lower them in front of your body to about a 45-degree angle so your body makes the shape of a banana.

**TIPS AND TRICKS**

- Don't sink in your hips; remain lifted and stable in your core and stack your hips.
- Don't forget to engage your inner thighs; as your top leg lowers to your bottom leg, squeeze your inner thighs and lengthen your top leg longer than your bottom heel.

**POSITION 1:** Inhale to lift the right leg to the ceiling (your knee faces up as your toes stretch to the ceiling).

## THE PAYOFF:

Tones and tightens your inner thighs.

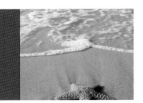

# Side Passé

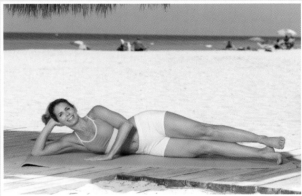

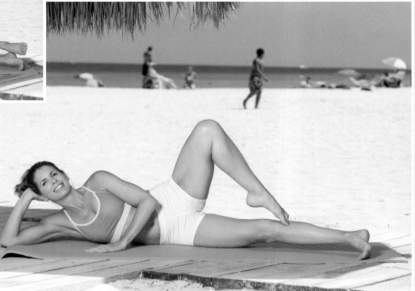

**STARTING POSITION:** Lie on your right side with your legs straight; your ankles, knees and hip bones stacked on top of one another; and your feet in a Pilates "V." Prop your head up with your right arm and then place your left arm, palm down, on the mat in front of your torso; relax your shoulders. Lift both legs at the same time and lower them in front of your body to about a 45-degree angle so your body makes the shape of a banana.

## TIPS AND TRICKS

- Don't sit back in your hips; if your hips are tight, it may be hard to open them, causing you to sit back. Focus on lifting your knee to the ceiling to open and stretch your hips; however, you don't have to lift your leg as high.

- Don't forget to engage your inner thighs and lift up from your pelvic floor to get lots more work.

**POSITION 1:** Inhale to bend your left leg so your knee lifts toward the ceiling, then slide your toes along the inside of your bottom leg.

## THE PAYOFF:

Takes inches off your thighs.

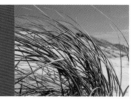

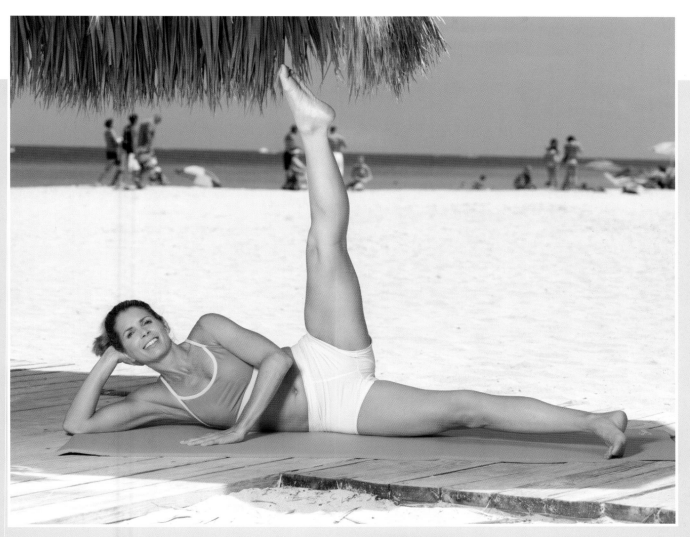

**POSITION 2:** Continue inhaling as the top leg lengthens to the ceiling. Exhale to lower your leg to the bottom leg—imagine one, two, three miles long—as the top heel extends past your bottom foot. Repeat three times, and then reverse the direction of the passé for three more.

# Single Leg Circle (front and back)

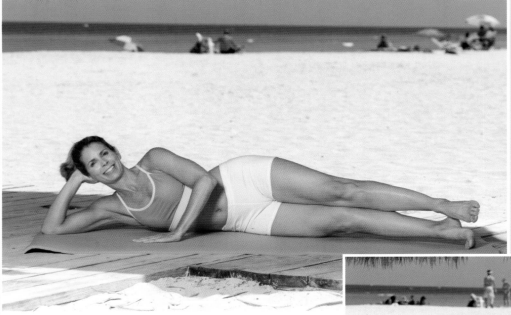

**STARTING POSITION:** Lie on your right side with your legs straight; your ankles, knees, and hip bones stacked on top of one another; and your feet in a Pilates "V." Prop your head up with your right arm and then place your left arm, palm down, on the mat in front of your torso; relax your shoulders. Lift both legs at the same time and lower them in front of your body to about a 45-degree angle so your body makes the shape of a banana. Lift your top leg to hip-height so it's parallel to the floor.

## TIPS AND TRICKS

- Don't move your hips as your leg circles; engage your booty and core to keep your hips stacked on top of each other.
- Keep your circles small at first if you still can't stabilize your hips.

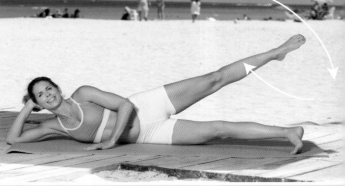

**POSITION 1:** Then circle the leg in front— your heels touch (or kiss) with every circle to engage your inner thighs. After 10 circles, reverse directions. Breathe normally.

## THE PAYOFF:

Takes inches off your legs and de-dimples, too.

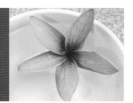

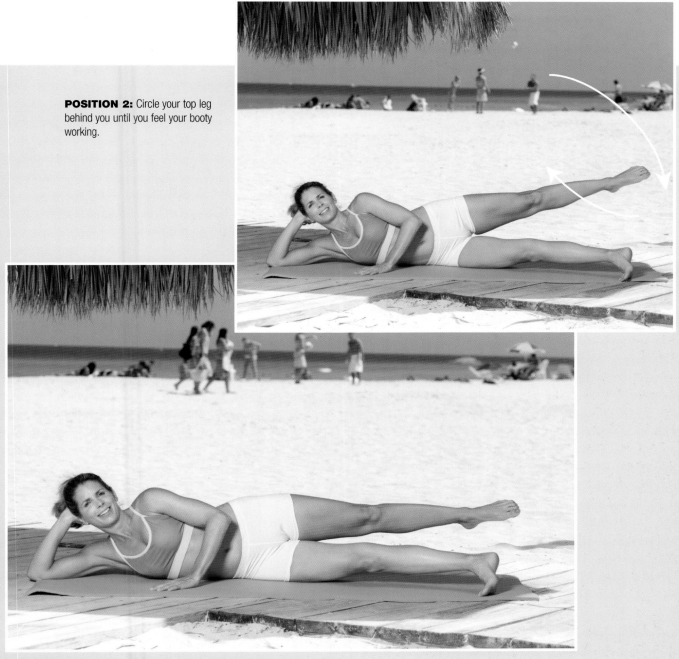

**POSITION 2:** Circle your top leg behind you until you feel your booty working.

**POSITION 3:** Circle the leg back. Keep your hips stacked on top of one another to engage your belly muscles. After 10 circles, reverse directions.

# Outer Thigh Lift

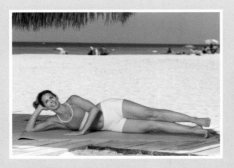

**STARTING POSITION:** Lie on your right side with your legs straight; your ankles, knees, and hip bones stacked on top of one another; and your feet in a Pilates "V." Prop your head up with your right arm and then place your left arm, palm down, on the mat in front of your torso; relax your shoulders. Lift both legs at the same time and lower them in front of your body to about a 45-degree angle, and then move your top leg behind you, with your toes parallel.

## TIPS AND TRICKS

- Don't move your hips; your hips remain stacked and stable as you lower and lift your leg.
- Don't lift too high; your goal is to focus on the outer thigh while also keeping your abs active.

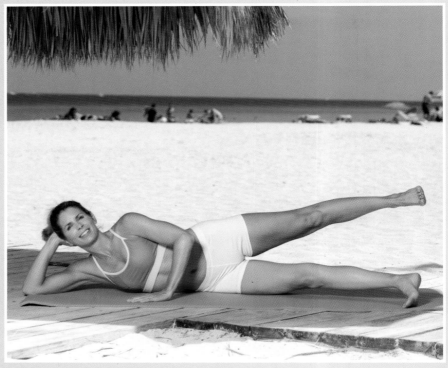

**POSITION 1:** : Inhale to lift your top leg to hip height and behind you so it's parallel to the floor, and then exhale to lower your legs to the floor. Breathe normally.

## THE PAYOFF:

Fights cellulite and takes inches off your thighs.

# Straight Line Leg Lift

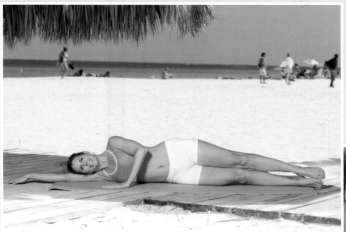

**STARTING POSITION:** Lie on your right side with your legs straight; your ankles, knees, and hip bones stacked on top of one another; and your feet parallel. Straighten your right arm and lower your head to rest on it.

**TIPS AND TRICKS**

- Don't strain to lift your legs; engage your core and lengthen your legs out from your torso.

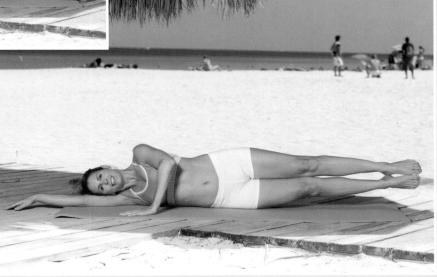

**POSITION 1:** Inhale to lift both legs just about an inch (2.5 cm) off the ground, then exhale to lower your legs to the floor.

## THE PAYOFF:

Fights cellulite and defines your waist.

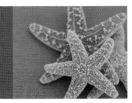

# Outer Thigh Lift, Close the Hatch, and Pac-Man

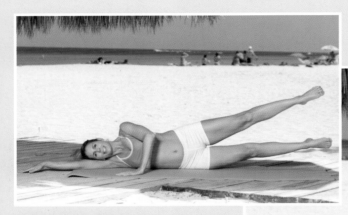

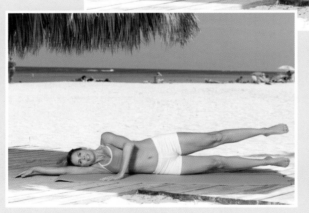

**STARTING POSITION:** For the Outer Thigh Lift, lie on your right side with your legs straight; your ankles, knees, and hip bones stacked on top of one another; your feet parallel; and your legs lifted off the ground. Straighten your right arm and lower your head to rest on it. Inhale to lift your top leg.

**TIPS AND TRICKS**

- Use your pelvic floor muscles to get extra booty benefits.

**POSITION 1:** Exhale to lower your top leg to your bottom leg.

**POSITION 2:** To Close the Hatch, inhale to lower your bottom leg to the floor.

## THE PAYOFF:

Gives you slim and sexy thighs.

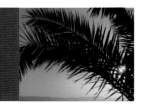

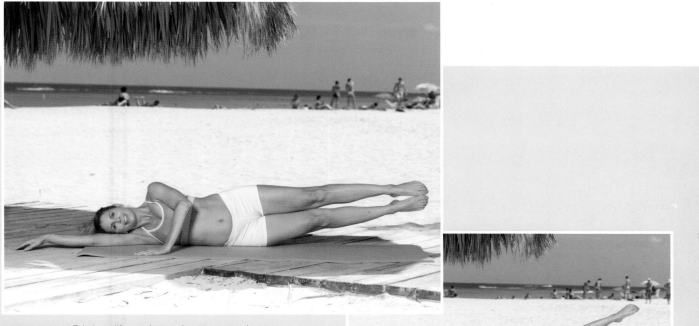

**POSITION 3:** Exhale to lift your bottom leg to your top leg.

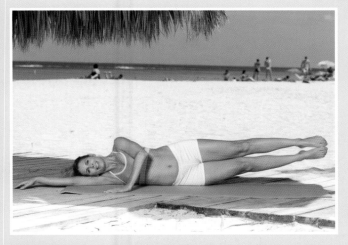

**POSITION 4:** For the Pac-Man: in the starting position or with your body in a straight line, inhale to open both of your legs very wide.

**POSITION 5:** Exhale to close them so you end up in a straight line for yummy outer and inner thigh work.

# Scissor Legs

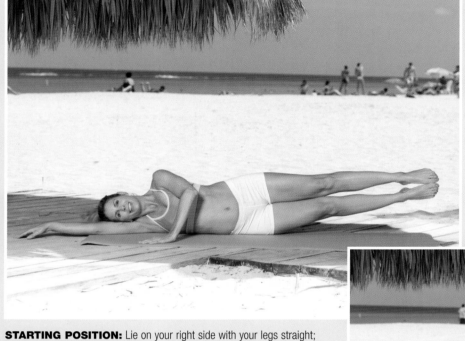

**STARTING POSITION:** Lie on your right side with your legs straight; your ankles, knees, and hip bones stacked on top of one another; and your feet parallel. Straighten your right arm and lower your head to rest on it. Lift both legs off the floor.

**TIPS AND TRICKS**

- Don't bend your knees; keep your legs straight to work your booty.
- Imagine a thin piece of glass between your legs, so you're holding your legs slightly apart.

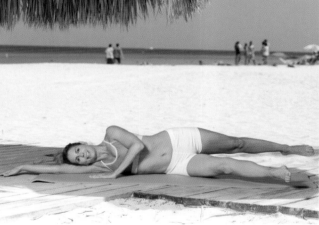

**POSITION 1:** Inhale to open your legs as wide as you can like a pair of scissors.

## THE PAYOFF:

Takes inches off your waist and gives mega booty benefits.

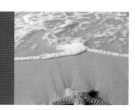

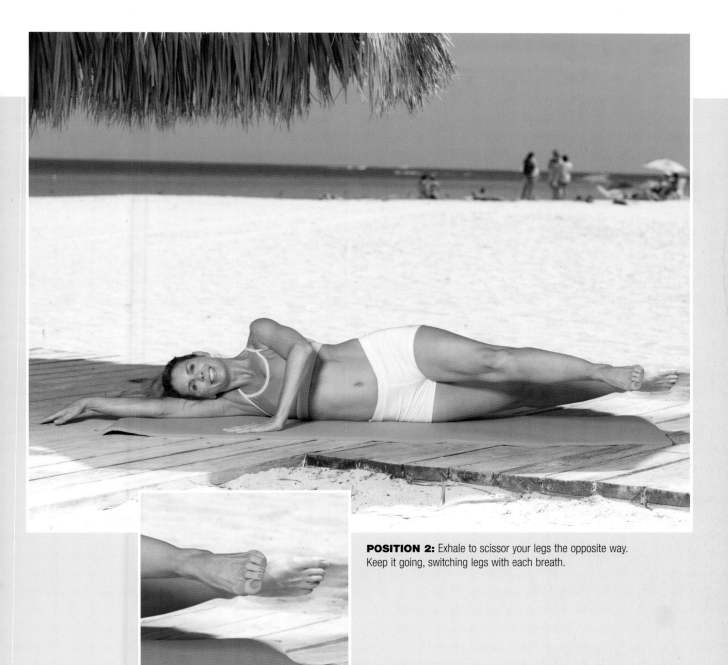

**POSITION 2:** Exhale to scissor your legs the opposite way. Keep it going, switching legs with each breath.

# Hot Potato

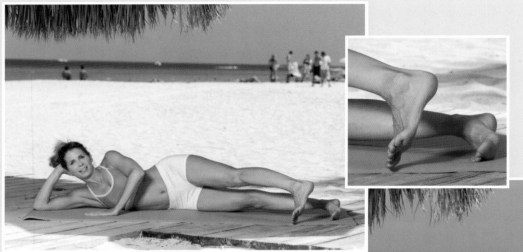

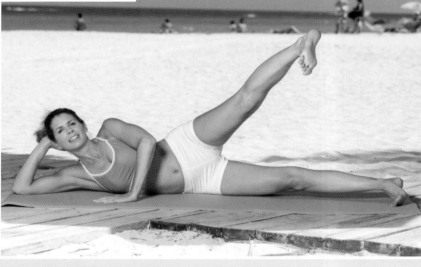

**STARTING POSITION:** Lie on your right side with your legs straight; your ankles, knees, and hip bones stacked on top of one another; and your feet in a Pilates "V." Prop your head up with your right arm and then place your left arm, palm down, on the mat in front of your torso; relax your shoulders. Lift both legs at the same time and lower them in front of your body to about a 45-degree angle. Lift the top leg and turn your toes under.

**TIPS AND TRICKS**

- Don't move your hips; keep them stacked using your abs.

**POSITION 1:** Inhale to lift your left leg to the ceiling. Exhale to lower your toes to the floor, as if you were dipping them in hot water; dip your toes 5 times in front.

## THE PAYOFF:

Develops sexy, slimmer thighs and underbutt.

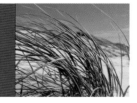

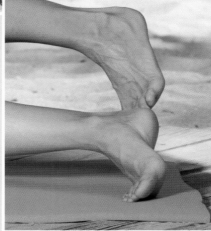

**POSITION 2:** Inhale to lift your top leg behind your bottom leg; lift as high as you can. Exhale to lower your toes behind you to the floor; dip your toes 5 times back. Lift leg as high as you can and repeat 3 times in front and then 3 times in back, then 1 time in front and 1 time in back.

# Clam

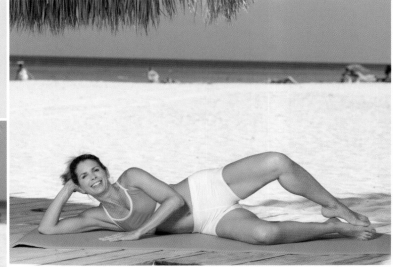

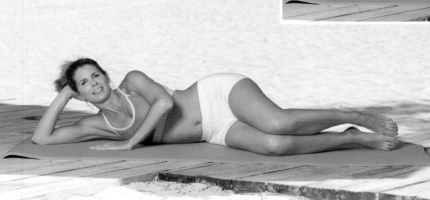

**POSITION 1:** Inhale to lift the top leg to the ceiling, keeping your knees stacked. Exhale to lower your leg.

**STARTING POSITION:** Lie on your right side with your knees bent and place them in front of your torso so your ankles, knees, and hip bones are stacked. Prop your head up with your right arm and then place your left arm, palm down, on the mat in front of your torso; relax your shoulders.

## TIPS AND TRICKS

- Don't lift too high; you should feel this work in the outer thigh. If you lift too high, you may miss out on the juicy outer thigh work.

## THE PAYOFF:

Seriously tightens, tones, and de-dimples your hips.

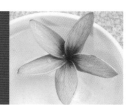

# two

# Froggy

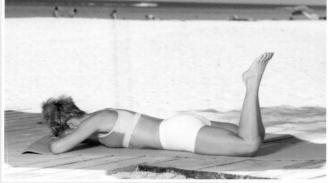

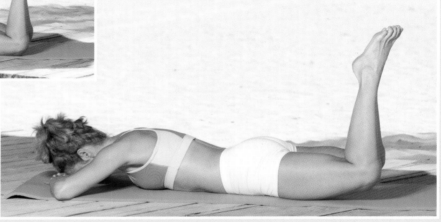

**STARTING POSITION:** Lie on your belly with your knees bent; place your hands under your head and cross them at the wrists, so your elbows are out to the sides. Rest your head on your hands. Open your knees so you can comfortably touch your heels—imagine putting a dime between your heels.

**TIPS AND TRICKS**

- Don't sag your belly; gently lift your belly to your spine to support your lower back.

- Don't strain your lower back; try readjusting your body by following the principles of extension (see sidebar). If it still hurts, stop and check with your doctor.

- Don't tense up; relax your shoulders, neck, and upper back.

**POSITION 1:** Inhale to lift your knees about an inch or two off the ground, and then exhale to lower them.

---

⭐ **GOOD BODY FORM IN EXTENSION**

To work safely in a back extension in the Froggy and Beat on the Belly (p. 98) exercises, review these tips:

- Your pubic bone and your two hip bones are your boney landmarks. You should feel those three points on the mat.

- Firm up your fanny and hamstrings the whole time to protect your lower back.

- Lift your belly button to your spine to provide support for your lower back.

- Relax your upper back.

---

## THE PAYOFF:

Fights cellulite on your butt.

# Beat on the Belly

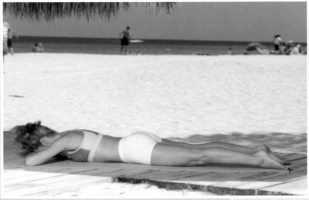

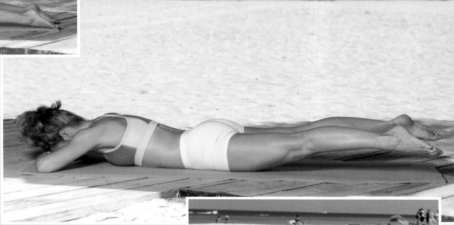

**STARTING POSITION:** Lie on your belly and straighten your legs long from your core. Place your hands under your head and cross them at the wrists, so your elbows are out to the sides. Rest your head on your hands. Lift your belly button to your spine.

## TIPS AND TRICKS

- Don't sag your belly; gently lift your belly to your spine to support your lower back.
- Don't strain your lower back; try readjusting your body by following the principles of extension (see sidebar on p. 96). If it still hurts, stop and check with your doctor.
- Don't tense up; relax your shoulders, neck, and upper back.
- Use your pelvic floor muscles and inner thighs to get extra booty work.

**POSITION 1:** Lift your legs about 2 to 3 inches (5 to 8 cm) off the mat.

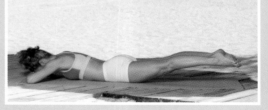

**POSITION 2:** Inhale to click and beat your heels together, counting to 5, then exhale as you beat your heels together for another set of 5. That's a total of 10 heel beats; your goal is 100 heel beats.

## THE PAYOFF:

Gives a speedy butt lift and a strong, fit back.

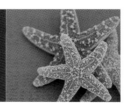

## THURSDAY: TURNING ON AND TONING UP WITH BODY BOOT CAMP

Today, repeat Monday's body boot camp, p. 65.

## FRIDAY: GETTING LEAN WITH CARDIO

Today, repeat Tuesday's cardio workout, p. 78.

## SATURDAY: USING PILATES FOR A SPEEDY BUTT LIFT

Today, repeat Wednesday's Pilates workout, p. 81.

## SUNDAY: LETTING GO!

Take today off, but make it count by introducing two more healthy eating habits. Try on your bikini, write down your comments, and keep going! You'll soon see the definition you're creating.

- **Eat exciting foods:** Eating the same colors day in and day out can translate to not getting a variety of precious nutrients. Put some colors: orange, blue, and yellow on your plate, starting with breakfast.

- **Focus on eating lean protein:** A strong bikini body needs fuel to keep going, so make sure you're eating lean protein, such as turkey, fish, chicken, and egg whites.

- **Don't be afraid of carbs:** All carbs are not bad; in fact, you need to refuel your body with good carbs, such as multigrain foods, rye, and whole wheat breads and the more seeds the better. How else will you get that bikini bod?

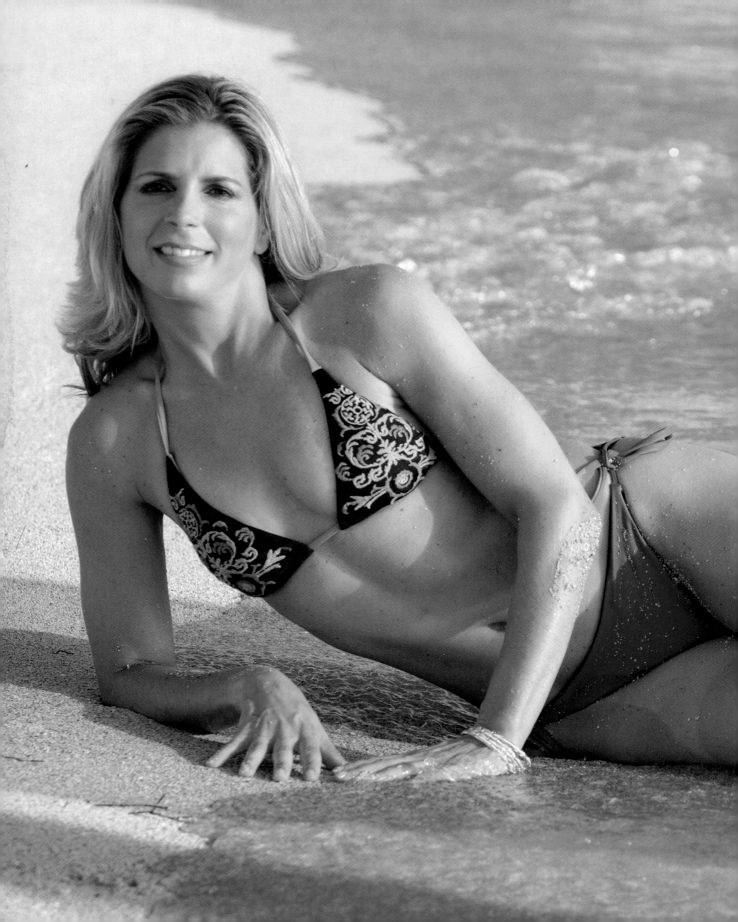

# week three

## GET A BEACH-BABE LOOK AND FLAT ABS

These exercises target everything that's good about a woman —her belly! No matter what you're thinking right now, you do have sexy abs, even if they're hidden. This week, you'll take inches (centimeters) off all over and uncover your sexy flat abs by focusing on your core muscles. You should have more strength and confidence, and yet you'll breathe a new lift into your core—and your attitude, well, it too will be hard-core.

**MONDAY**          Meeting the Cardio Challenge

**TUESDAY**         Getting an All Over Hard-Core Workout

**WEDNESDAY**       Meeting the Cardio Challenge

**THURSDAY**        Getting an All Over Hard-Core Workout

**FRIDAY**          Meeting the Cardio Challenge

**SATURDAY**        Showing Off Simply Gorgeous Abs with Pilates

**SUNDAY**          Taking It Easy–You're Worth It!

# week three

## M T W T

| MONDAY | TUESDAY | WEDNESDAY | THURSDAY |
|---|---|---|---|
| Meeting the Cardio Challenge | Getting an All Over Hard-Core Workout | Meeting the Cardio Challenge | Getting an All Over Hard-Core Workout |

| MONDAY | TUESDAY | WEDNESDAY | THURSDAY |
|---|---|---|---|
| **1**. 3 minutes: Warm up by walking 3.5 mph (5.5 kph), no grade<br><br>**2.** 8 minutes: Walk 3.5 to 4.0 mph (5.5 to 6.0 kph), 3-6 percent incline<br><br>**3.** 2 minutes: Run 5.5 to 6.0 mph (9.0 to 10.0 kph), 3-6 percent incline<br><br>**4.** Repeat steps 2 and 3 four more times<br><br>**5.** 2 minutes: Cool down by walking 3.0 to 3.5 mph (4.5 to 5.5 kph), no grade | **SET 1**<br>Squat with Overhead Press<br>Front Plank<br>Overhead Triceps Extension<br><br>**SET 2**<br>Walking Lunge<br>Right- and Left-Side Plank<br><br>**SET 3**<br>Reverse Lunge with Biceps Curls<br>Plank with Outer Thigh Lift<br>Push-ups | **1**. 3 minutes: Warm up by walking 3.5 mph (5.5 kph), no grade<br><br>**2.** 8 minutes: Walk 3.5 to 4.0 mph (5.5 to 6.0 kph), 3-6 percent incline<br><br>**3.** 2 minutes: Run 5.5 to 6.0 mph (9.0 to 10.0 kph), 3-6 percent incline<br><br>**4.** Repeat steps 2 and 3 four more times<br><br>**5.** 2 minutes: Cool down by walking 3.0 to 3.5 mph (4.5 to 5.5 kph), no grade | **SET 1**<br>Squat with Overhead Press<br>Front Plank<br>Overhead Triceps Extension<br><br>**SET 2**<br>Walking Lunge<br>Right- and Left-Side Plank<br><br>**SET 3**<br>Reverse Lunge with Biceps Curls<br>Plank with Outer Thigh Lift<br>Push-ups |

## FRIDAY

### Meeting
### the Cardio
### Challenge

**1**. 3 minutes: Warm up by
walking 3.5 mph
(5.5 kph), no grade

**2.** 8 minutes: Walk 3.5 to
4.0 mph (5.5 to 6.0 kph),
3-6 percent incline

**3.** 2 minutes: Run 5.5 to 6.0
mph (9.0 to 10.0 kph),
3-6 percent incline

**4.** Repeat steps 2 and 3 four
more times

**5.** 2 minutes: Cool down by
walking 3.0 to 3.5 mph
(4.5 to 5.5 kph), no grade

## SATURDAY

### Showing Off
### Simply Gorgeous
### Abs with Pilates

**The following are the
Pilates exercises you'll be
doing today:**

The Hundred

Roll-up

Roll Over

Single Leg Circle

Rolling Like a Ball

Single Leg Stretch

Double Leg Stretch

Straight Leg Scissors

Double Straight Leg Lift

Criss-Cross

Spine Stretch

Open Leg Rocker

Corkscrew

Saw

Swan

Single Leg Kick

Double Leg Kick

Neck Pull

Shoulder Bridge
    with One Leg

Teaser 2

The Seal

## SUNDAY

### Taking it Easy
### You're
### Worth It!

OFF

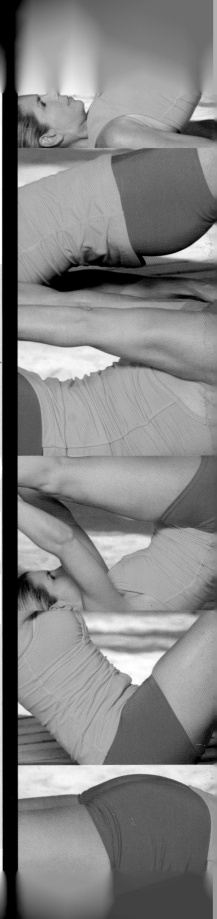

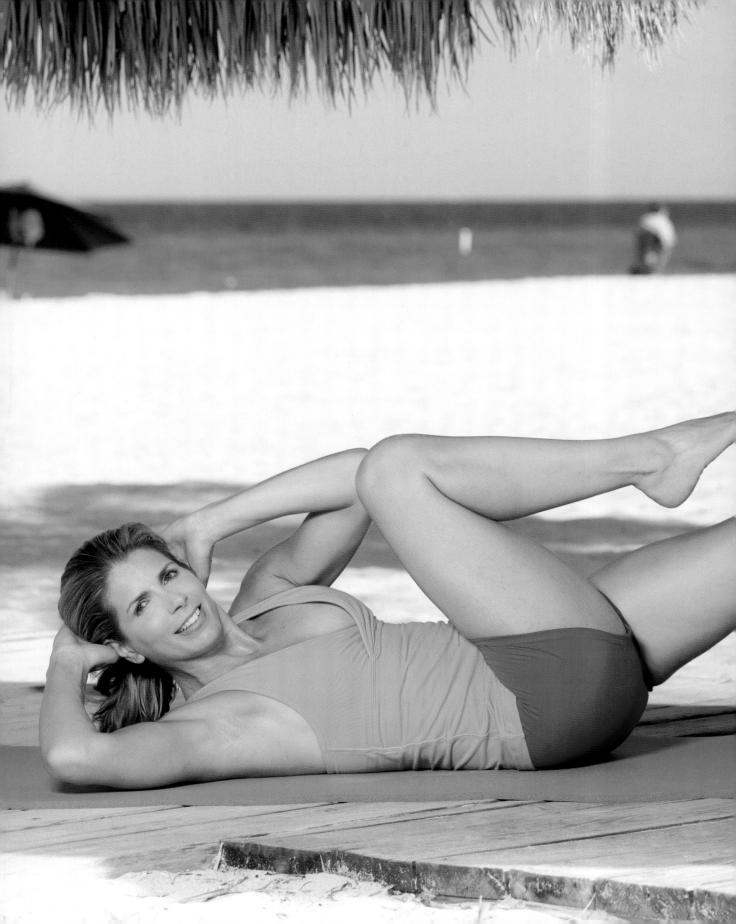

# MONDAY: MEETING THE CARDIO CHALLENGE

Today, you'll hit the treadmill. This week's goal is still three intense cardio-interval sessions, doing up to 50 to 55 minutes each, only now you'll increase the intensity with hills or inclines (no grade means no incline) To get lean and get a speedy butt lift, your inclines should be steep enough to really feel your butt and calves working. Remember, you're alternating between low intensity (recovery) and high intensity (choppy talk). If your recovery between intervals seems too short, you're running too fast. Your goal is to be breathless yet feel like you can talk a little, not carry on a full conversation. If you absolutely hate the treadmill, pick another cardio machine: stair stepper, elliptical trainer, or stationary bike, using the intensity scale in the introduction to this book of help you. If you don't have access to a cardio macine, you can walk, run, or bike outside using a hill as the incline.

Here's your treadmill workout:

1. 3 minutes: Warm up by walking 3.5 mph (5.5 kph), no grade

2. 8 minutes: Walk 3.5 to 4.0 mph (5.5 to 6.0 kph), 3-6 percent incline (breathless pace)

3. 2 minutes: Run 5.5 to 6.0 mph (9.0 to 10.0 kph), 3-6 percent incline (choppy talk pace)

4. Repeat steps 2 and 3 four more times

5. 2 minutes: Cool down by walking 3.0 to 3.5 mph (4.5 to 5.5 kph), no grade

# TUESDAY: GETTING AN ALL OVER HARD-CORE WORKOUT

Some of these exercises may look familiar, but now they get a fresh twist to help you get more sexy muscles and flat abs out of every rep. You'll need a couple sets of dumbbells: 15 to 20 pounds (7 to 9 kg) for your legs and a lighter pair, 8 to 10 pounds (4 to 5 kg) for your arms.

To do this all over workout you'll do Set 1 three times, doing 15 to 20 reps of each exercise in that set, and then repeat that set two more times. For example, complete 15 to 20 slow and controlled reps of each exercise unless I tell you differently: Squat with Overhead Press, Front Plank (hold for 30 to 60 seconds), and Overhead Triceps Extension. Repeat that set two times before moving on to Set 2, and then finish with Set 3. Total time should be about 45 minutes to 1 hour. If you're not clear on what a set or a rep is, flip to the introduction of this book. And don't forget to warm up on the treadmill for 5 minutes at 3.5 mph (5.5 kph) before beginning.

**SET 1**

Squat with Overhead Press

Front Plank

Overhead Triceps Extension

**SET 2**

Walking Lunge

Right- and Left-Side Plank

**SET 3**

Reverse Lunge with Biceps Curls

Plank with Outer Thigh Lift

Push-ups

## BREATH WORK

Just about every move in this workout strengthens your core, so use your Pilates breath to get more core activation (see the introduction for details). Exhale deeply to shrink your waistline, pulling your belly button toward spine to support your lower back. In other words, scoop—no bulgy belly!

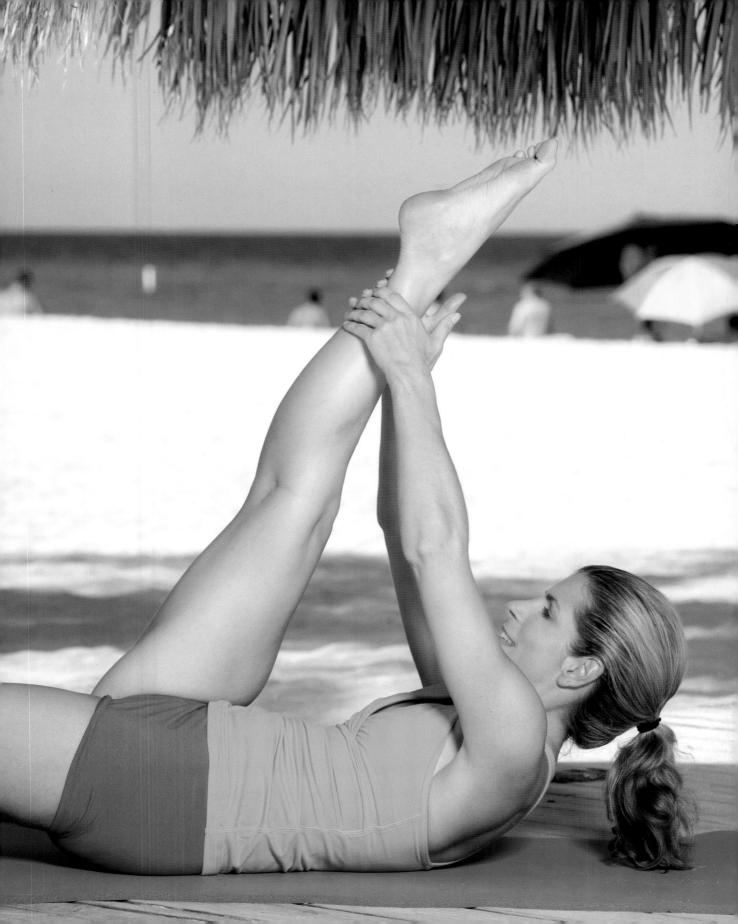

# Squat with Overhead Press

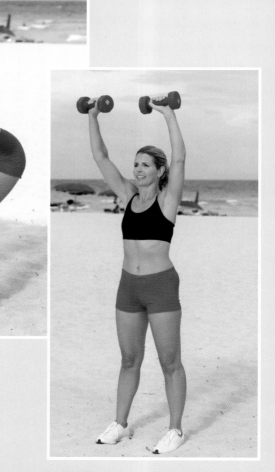

**STARTING POSITION:** In a squat position, with your thighs about parallel to the floor, knees aligned over your second and third toes, hold an 8- to 10-pound (4 to 5 kg) dumbbell in each hand. Bend your elbows so the dumbbells are just above your shoulders, keeping your knuckles up. Look forward or slightly up.

## TIPS AND TRICKS

- Don't lean forward; your torso will naturally come forward slightly as you squat. If you want extra butt work, sit back on your heels so your hips and knees are parallel to the floor.

- Don't turn your knees in; keep your knees stable as you squat, and then pivot into a lunge.

- Don't forget your sexy posture; your torso is straight up and your shoulders are relaxed, your chin is up, and your toes point forward.

- Don't arch your lower back; engage your abdominals during the entire movement to provide support for your lower back.

**POSITION 1:** In one motion, stand up and press your dumbbells towards the ceiling. Repeat 15 to 20 reps.

## THE PAYOFF:

Overhauls your butt, legs, and core.

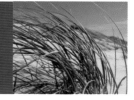

# Front Plank
REPLAY WEEK FOUR

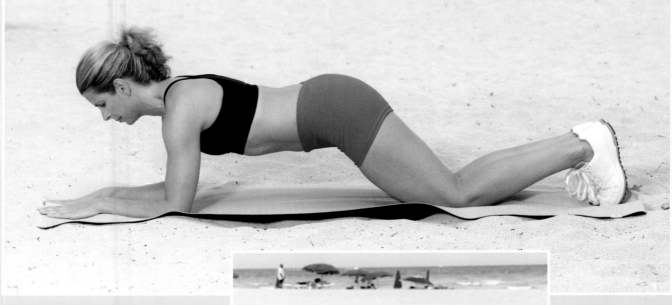

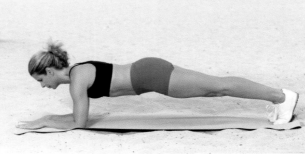

**STARTING POSITION:** On your knees, place your elbows directly under your shoulders, palms down. With your toes curled under, place your heels together.

**TIPS AND TRICKS**

- Don't sag your belly; gently lift your belly button toward your spine to strengthen your core while giving your lower back support.

- Don't forget to firm up your fanny, inner thighs, and pelvic floor; oh-so-much power is wasted if you don't use them!

- Don't elevate your shoulders; draw your shoulder blades down your back to engage your upper back.

- Don't drop your head; gaze at the floor as you lengthen from the top of your head.

**POSITION 1:** Lift your legs, pelvis, and torso off the floor in one motion. Balance on your toes and elbows, keeping your back perfectly straight; imagine that everything from your head to your heels is like steel. Hold for 30 to 60 seconds, and then do 2 more reps.

## THE PAYOFF:

Sculpts all over and strengthens your core.

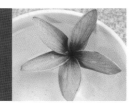

# Overhead Triceps Extension

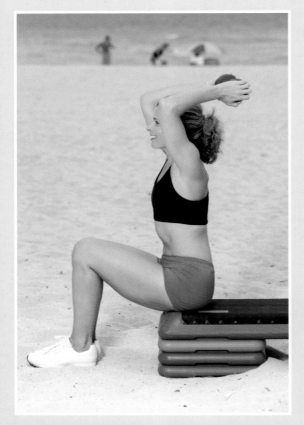

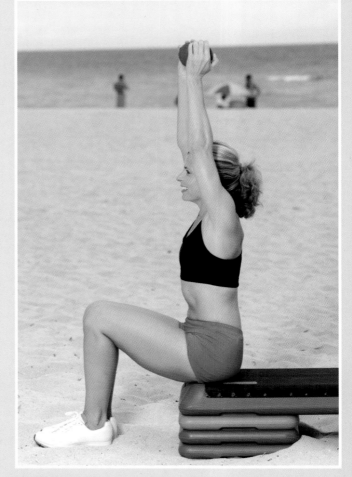

**STARTING POSITION:** Sit on a bench or stand and hold an 8- to 10-pound (4 to 5 kg) dumbbell in your hands. Lift your arms over your head and bend your arms so the dumbbell is behind your head, keeping your shoulders down.

**TIPS AND TRICKS**

- Don't round your spine; keep your abs active and lengthen from the top of your head.
- Don't let your shoulders lift toward your ears; try to relax your upper back.

**POSITION 1:** Straighten your arms to the ceiling, leading with your knuckles. Keep your upper arms still so you can fully extend your arms. Do 15 to 20 reps.

## THE PAYOFF:

Lets you say good-bye to flabby arms.

# Walking Lunge

## REPLAY WEEK TWO

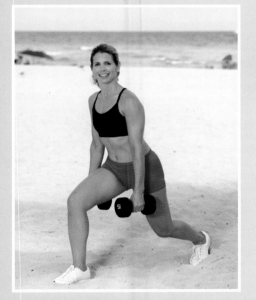

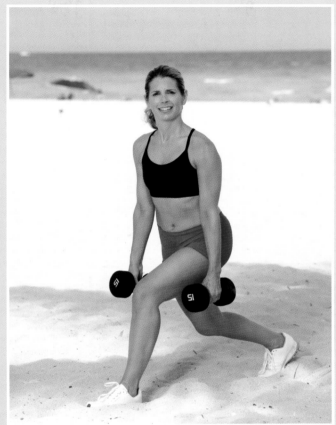

**STARTING POSITION:** Stand with your feet hip width apart and hold a pair of 15- to 20-pound (7 to 9 kg) dumbbells. You'll need enough room to walk about 20 steps. Step forward with your right foot to lower your body in a lunge so your right thigh is parallel to the floor while your left thigh is perpendicular to the floor (your knee should almost touch the floor).

### TIPS AND TRICKS

- Don't lean forward; align your knee over your second and third toes, keeping your body weight in the lunge leg.

- Don't round your spine; keep your chest lifted, your shoulders relaxed, and your toes pointing forward.

- Use your abs to support your lower back.

**POSITION 1:** Walk your left foot up to your right foot, come to a standing position, and then lunge forward with your left leg. Keep your spine straight and lifted as you walk. Do 15 to 20 reps.

## THE PAYOFF:

There's nothing better for your legs, butt, and abs.

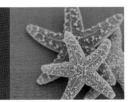

# Right- and Left-Side Plank

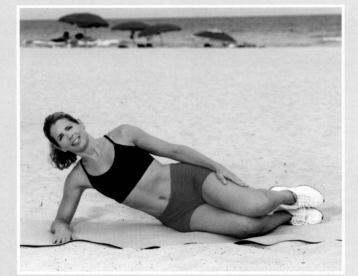

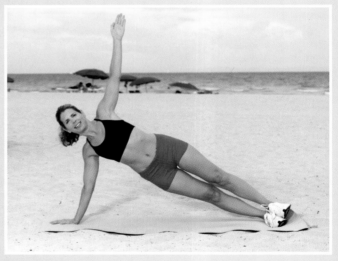

**POSITION 1:** Lift your torso, hips, and legs off the floor in one motion. Balance on your right hand and on the right leading edge of your foot, stacking your feet on top of one another.

**STARTING POSITION:** Sit on your right side with your knees slightly pulled into your body, stacking your knees on top of one another. Place your hand on the floor slightly away from your shoulder.

## TIPS AND TRICKS

- Don't droop your torso in the middle; focus on your breath work and lift your trunk to the ceiling.
- Don't hang in your wrist; your wrist should line up under your shoulder and lift, lift, lift!
- If you can't maintain good form, do this plank on your elbows as shown in position 1 of Plank with Outer Thigh Lift (p. 114).

**POSITION 2:** Lift your left arm to the ceiling, forming a "T" shape with your body. Repeat 3 times, holding for 15 seconds, and then switch sides.

## THE PAYOFF:

Takes inches off your waist and uncovers your sexy abs.

# Reverse Lunge with Biceps Curls

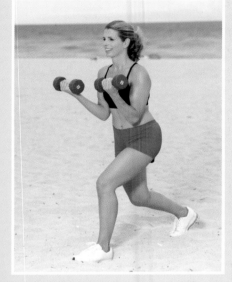

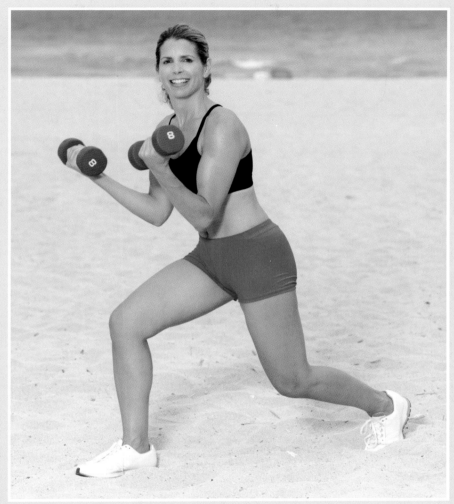

**STARTING POSITION:** Stand with your legs together and hold an 8- to 10-pound (4 to 5 kg) dumbbell in each hand with your arms straight by your sides.

## TIPS AND TRICKS

- Don't lean forward; align your knee over your second and third toes, keeping your body weight in the lunge leg.

- Don't round your spine; keep your chest lifted, shoulders relaxed, and toes pointing forward.

- Use your abs to support your lower back.

- Don't swing your arms; curl with control and keep your arms within its natural alignment of your shoulders.

**POSITION 1:** Lunge back with your left foot so your right knee bends at a 90-degree angle, with your knee over your toes, while curling your dumbbells up toward your chest. Do 12 reps on each leg, alternating legs.

## THE PAYOFF:

Boosts your bottom line and leans out your arms.

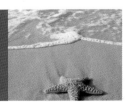

# Plank with Outer Thigh Lift

REPLAY WEEK FOUR

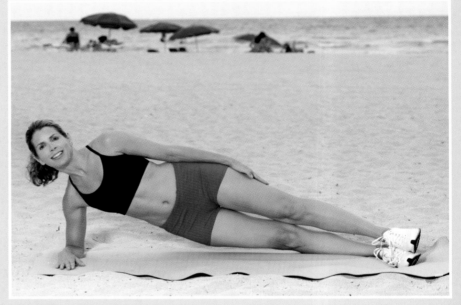

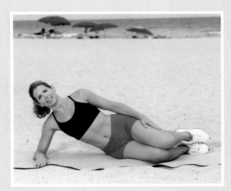

**STARTING POSITION:** Sit on your right side with your knees slightly pulled into your body, stacking your knees on top of one another. Place your elbow on the floor slightly out from your shoulder, fingertips away from your torso.

### TIPS AND TRICKS

- Don't droop your torso; focus on your breath work and lift your torso to the ceiling.
- Don't hang in your neck or shoulders as you lift your leg. Just don't lower and lift, hold the leg up until you have enough strength to maintain good form.

**POSITION 1:** Lift your torso, hips, and legs off the floor in one motion. Balance on your right elbow and on the right leading edge of your foot, stacking your feet on top of one another.

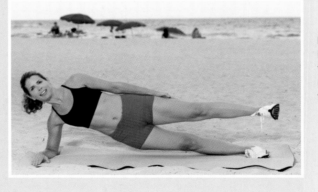

**POSITION 2:** Lift your top leg up toward the ceiling and then lower it to the plank (bottom leg). Repeat 5 to 8 times, and then switch sides.

## THE PAYOFF:

Sculpts all over and de-dimples your thighs.

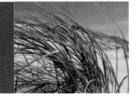

# Push-ups
## REPLAY WEEK FOUR

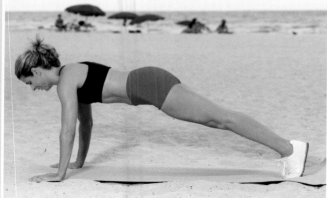

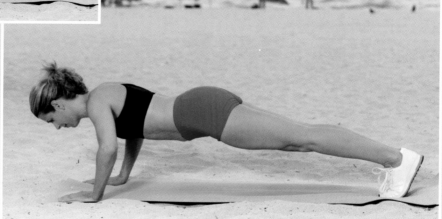

**STARTING POSITION:** On your knees, place your hands on the floor directly under your shoulders, palms down. With your toes curled under, place your heels together and lift your legs, pelvis, and torso off the floor in one motion. Balance on your toes and elbows, keeping your back perfectly straight, imagining that everything from your head to your heels is like steel.

### TIPS AND TRICKS

- Don't sag your belly; gently lift your belly button toward your spine to strengthen your core while giving your lower back support.

- Don't forget to firm up your fanny, inner thighs, and pelvic floor; oh-so-much power is wasted if you don't use them!

- Don't elevate your shoulders; draw your shoulder blades down your back to engage your upper back, and don't lower your torso too much.

- Don't drop your head; look at the floor as you lengthen from the top of your head.

**POSITION 1:** Bend your elbows at the sides to lower your body to the floor. Push up to starting position. Do 15 to 20 reps.

## THE PAYOFF:

Sculpts all over and develops a beautiful chest.

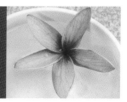

# WEDNESDAY: MEETING THE CARDIO CHALLENGE

Today, repeat Monday's cardio challenge, p.105.

# THURSDAY: GETTING AN ALL OVER HARD-CORE WORKOUT

Today, repeat Tuesday's hard-core workout, p.106.

# FRIDAY: MEETING THE CARDIO CHALLENGE

Today, repeat Monday's cardio challenge, p.105.

# SATURDAY: SHOWING OFF SIMPLY GORGEOUS ABS WITH PILATES

You've probably been doing just fine, even if you feel a little overwhelmed. After all, you're moving through lots of exercises. In Pilates, you learn by going over it and over it. Some of my students have been training with me for several years, and I still get an "Ah-ha, now I feel it!" sensation now and then. Keep at it, especially if you want simply gorgeous abs!

Your Pilates routine is basically the same as week one, but now we're adding on some intensity. Follow the exercises in the order shown, and follow all directions, including the breathing patterns. Remember to scoop your abs to your spine the whole time—no bulgy belly! Don't forget to run through your mental and verbal checklist, head, neck, shoulders, and hips (see the introduction for details), as you do the following sequence of exercises:

- The Hundred
- Roll-up
- Roll Over
- Single Leg Circle
- Rolling Like a Ball
- Single Leg Stretch
- Double Leg Stretch
- Straight Leg Scissors
- Double Straight Leg Lift
- Criss-Cross
- Spine Stretch
- Open Leg Rocker
- Corkscrew
- Saw
- Swan
- Single Leg Kick
- Double Leg Kick
- Neck Pull
- Shoulder Bridge with One Leg
- Teaser 2
- The Seal

Even if you're carrying a little winter "insulation" around your middle and feel not-so-sexy in those sweats, get off the couch and onto the mat. You'll feel sexier because you're doing something healthy for your body. Remember, your best abs, thighs, and butt are just inches away. Don't stop—you're worth it!

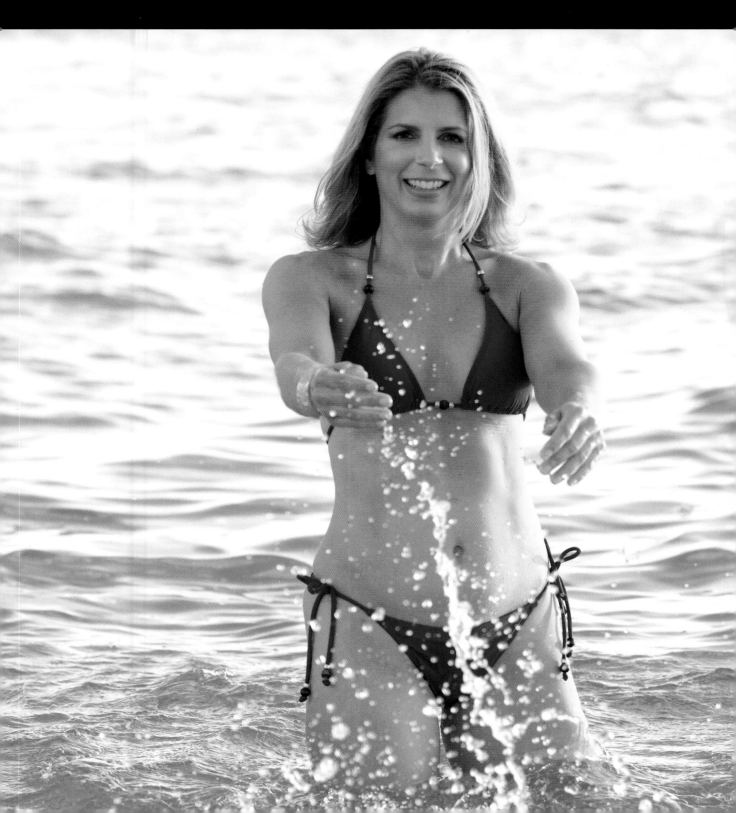

# The Hundred

REPLAY WEEKS ONE, TWO, FOUR, FIVE, SIX

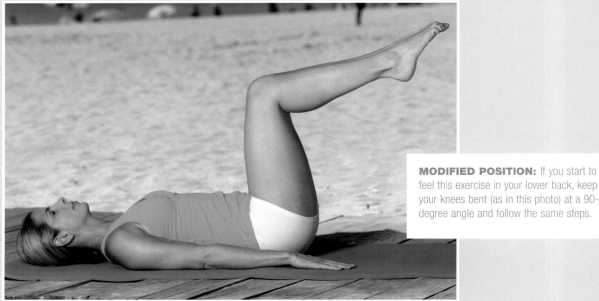

**MODIFIED POSITION:** If you start to feel this exercise in your lower back, keep your knees bent (as in this photo) at a 90-degree angle and follow the same steps.

**STARTING POSITION:** Lie on your back with your knees bent, feet hip width apart. Lengthen your arms by your sides, palms down.

**TIPS AND TRICKS**

- Don't bounce your torso as your arms move up and down; focus on your exhale to engage your abs, belly button to spine.

- Don't gasp for breath; keep it flowing from inhale to exhale; it's okay if you can't make it to a count of 5, do what you can.

- Don't tense your neck or clench your jaw; relax, neck tension is so not sexy! If you feel any strain, put a hand behind your head for support. Remember, strong abs can help lift your head. When they're weak, you may feel tension in your neck. Do what you can, but always protect your neck. Rest if you need it!

- Don't let your lower back come off the mat; melt your spine to the mat, using your abs to protect your lower back.

## THE PAYOFF:

Leads to sexy, strong abs and a killer figure.

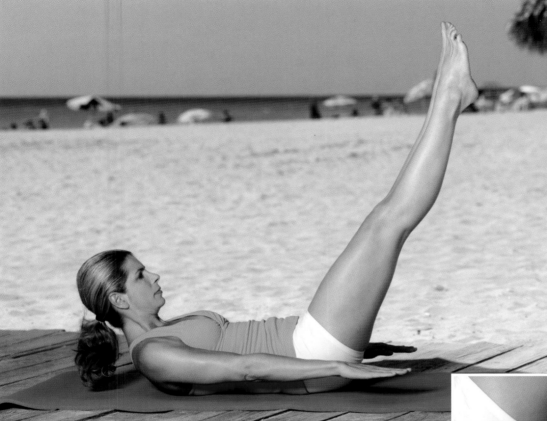

**POSITION 1:** In one motion, straighten your legs to the ceiling, feet in the Pilates "V." Curl your chin to your chest to lift your shoulders off the floor, keep your neck long. Lift and lengthen your arms past your hips, palms down, and begin pumping your arms by your sides.

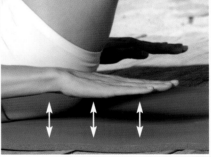

**POSITION 2:** Keeping your wrists straight, inhale to stretch your fingertips long, and pump your arms about 6 to 8 inches (15 to 20 cm) off the floor, as if you're moving your arms through thick molasses, for a count of 5, and then exhale for 5 breaths, emptying your lungs completely to drop your abs to your spine. This completes one breath cycle. Complete 10 breath cycles, thus adding up to The Hundred.

# Roll-up

REPLAY WEEKS ONE, TWO, FOUR

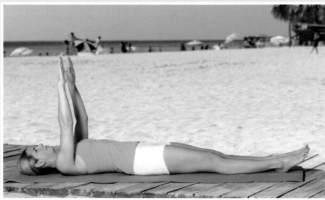

**STARTING POSITION:** Lie on your back with your legs straight, feet in Pilates "V." Straighten your arms so your fingertips reach to the ceiling. Drop the backs of your shoulders against the mat, and slide your shoulder blades down your back.

### TIPS AND TRICKS

- Don't lift your shoulders to your ears; instead, drop your armpits to your hips.
- Don't jerk up; if you can't roll up in a controlled motion, bend your knees and grab the backs of your thighs to help you.
- Don't plop down; control is crucial, so try rolling down as you press your heels away from your hips. Stay heavy in your heinie!
- Don't forget to squeeze your inner thighs. Place a rolled-up hand towel between your legs to work your inner thighs.
- Don't crane your neck; look at your belly to keep your head in line with your spine the whole time.

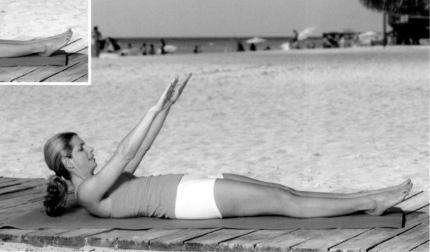

**POSITION 1:** Inhale to curl your chin to your chest, lifting the backs of your shoulders off the mat to look between your arms-keep your neck long. Peel your spine off the mat as if it were a string of pearls.

## THE PAYOFF:

Develops strong, flat abs and a flexible, healthy spine.

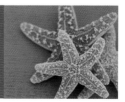

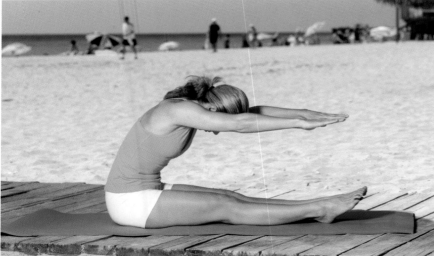

**POSITION 2:** Exhale to round over, scooping your abs to your spine. Reach your fingers past your toes and flex your feet to stretch your hamstrings.

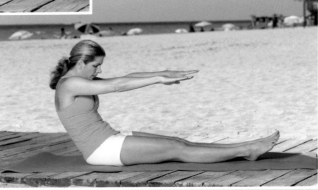

**POSITION 3:** Inhale to lift your pubic bone toward the ceiling, scooping your abs.

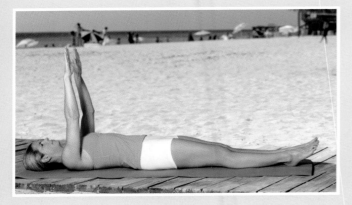

**POSITION 4:** Exhale to roll down, vertebra by vertebra, to the starting position. Repeat 3 to 5 times.

# Roll Over

REPLAY WEEKS FOUR, FIVE, SIX

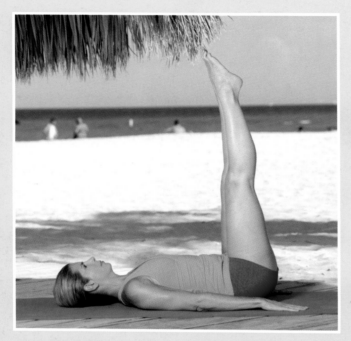

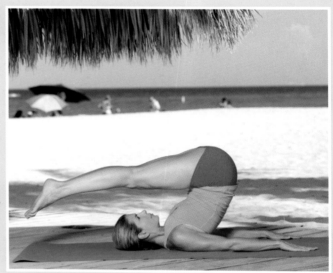

**STARTING POSITION:** Lie on your back with your legs straight at a 90-degree angle, feet in a Pilates "V." Straighten your arms by your sides, lengthening your fingertips. Slide your shoulder blades down your back.

## TIPS AND TRICKS

- Inhale to lift your legs over your head; exhale to lower your legs.

- Don't do this exercise if you have a neck or upper back injury. In addition, if you have high blood pressure or a condition called macular degeneration, check with your doctor. Exercises on your head, neck, and shoulders may not be appropriate for you.

- Don't plop down; roll down with control, pressing the backs of your arms into the mat and reaching your fingertips long to help you sink each bone into the mat.

- Don't lift your head off the mat as you roll down; scoop your abs to give you extra power.

**POSITION 1:** In one movement, press your palms into the mat and inhale to lift your hips over your head, keeping your legs closed. Hover your toes a few inches off the mat, keeping your knees directly over your eyes. Reach your fingertips long so the weight of your body doesn't land on your neck.

## THE PAYOFF:

Uncovers sexy abs and creates a fit and flexible spine

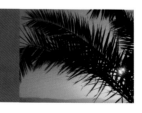

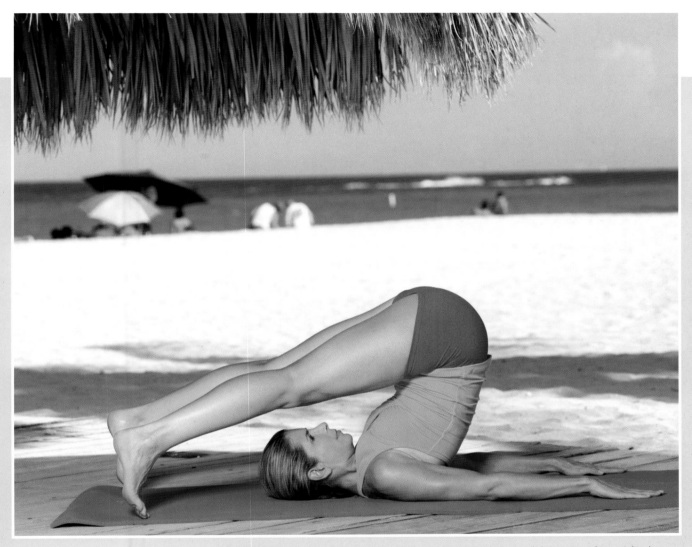

**POSITION 2:** Open your legs just past your shoulders and exhale to roll down your spine vertebra by vertebra. Feel each spinal bone pressing into the mat as you roll down until your sacrum, or the flat bone on your lower back, touches the mat. Do 3 reps with your legs closed and then 3 reps in the reverse direction, totaling 6 times. Imagine a string of pearls hitting the mat one at a time.

# Single Leg Circle

REPLAY WEEKS ONE, TWO, FOUR, FIVE, SIX

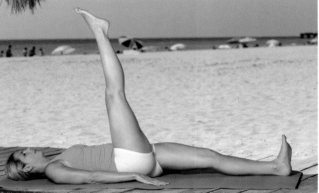

**POSITION 1:** Press your left heel into the mat and inhale to lift your right leg with toes pointing to your nose.

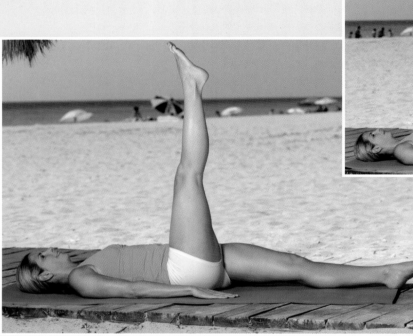

**STARTING POSITION:** Lie on your back with your left leg straight on the floor while your right leg is at a 90-degree angle, toes reaching long to the ceiling. Straighten your arms by your sides, palms down. Drop the backs of your shoulders against the mat, and slide your shoulder blades down your back.

**TIPS AND TRICKS**

- Don't rock your hips from side to side as the leg circles; fire up your core and keep your circles small at first.
- Press the palms of your hands, the backs of your arms, and the back of your head firmly into the mat, which will help stabilize you.
- Don't forget to exhale deeply to stabilize your torso and strengthen your abs.

## THE PAYOFF:

Develops sexy, flat abs and takes inches off your thighs.

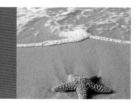

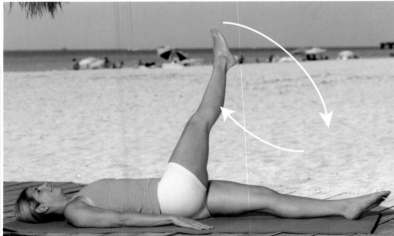

**POSITION 2:** Exhale to move the right leg across your body, inner thighs active.

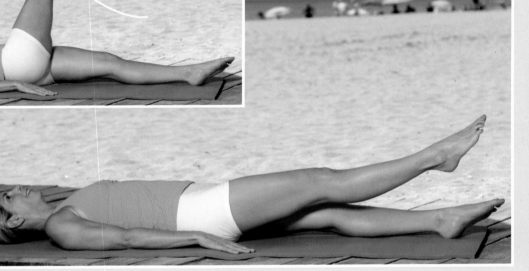

**POSITION 3:** Continue to exhale while moving your right leg to the opposite foot.

**POSITION 4:** Continue to exhale and circle your leg so it ends up at your nose. Inhale and pause slightly before circling your leg again. Imagine a string pulling your big toe to the ceiling to lengthen your leg as you circle it. Repeat 5 leg circles and then reverse the circle for 5. Repeat with the left leg.

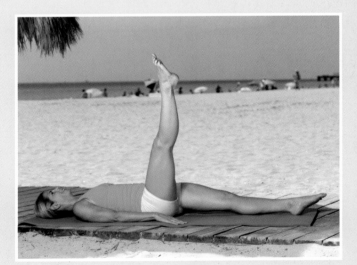

# Rolling Like a Ball

REPLAY WEEKS ONE, TWO, FOUR, FIVE, SIX

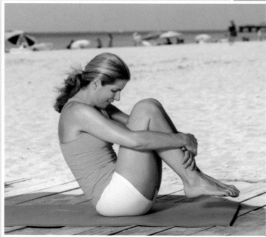

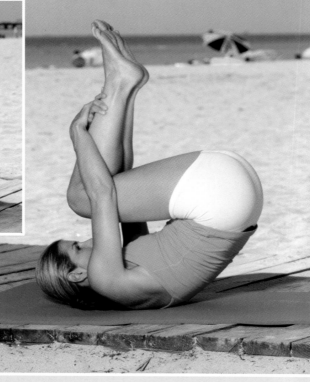

**STARTING POSITION:** Sit at the edge of the mat and slide your booty to your heels. Wrap your arms around your legs, elbows out to the sides. Place your hands on your shins, and cross them at the wrists. Your heels stay close to your bottom. Lower your head between your knees so your spine is rounded, belly button to your spine. Lift your toes off the floor, about 2 inches (5 cm). Use your belly muscles to balance.

## TIPS AND TRICKS

- Don't roll on your neck; it's about lifting your fanny to the ceiling and keeping active in your belly, so you roll only on your upper back.
- Don't lift your shoulders; instead, drop your armpits to your hips.

**POSITION 1:** Inhale to roll back to the middle portion of your back, scooping your abs and lifting your booty to the ceiling. Stay rounded so you don't roll back onto your head. Exhale to lift through your pelvic floor and scoop your abs for extra power to roll up and balance. Imagine you're a ball in motion. Repeat 8 to 10 times.

### ⭐ THE FIVES: BEST AB SERIES EVER

The Fives are done in order, one right after another, to challenge all your abdominal muscles. Right after the Single and Double Straight Leg Stretch, do Straight Leg Scissors, Double Leg Lift, and Criss-Cross. Don't rest in between exercises, challenge your belly to do more and more, and do 5 to 10 reps of each.

## THE PAYOFF:

Leads to a healthy, strong, and flexible spine.

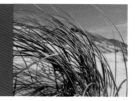

# Single Leg Stretch

REPLAY WEEKS ONE, TWO, FOUR

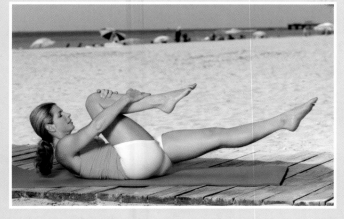

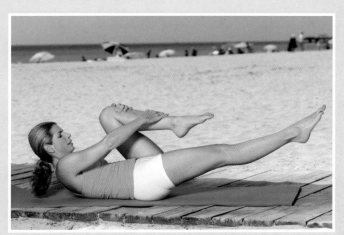

**STARTING POSITION:** Lie on your back with your knees to your chest. Place your right hand on the outside of your right shin and your left hand just below your knee, elbows out to your sides. In one motion, inhale to curl your chin to your chest to lift your shoulders off the ground and straighten your left leg so your toes are in line with your nose while giving your right knee two little hugs.

**TIPS AND TRICKS**

- Don't freak out about the hand placement; it keeps your knee in line with your ankle and hip, but if you get totally frustrated, just clasp your hands and place them behind your head for support.
- Don't rock from side to side while moving your legs; engage your abs to stay stable in your torso.
- Don't bend your knees; as you move your legs away from your torso, stretch them as far as possible.
- Don't look at the ceiling; look between your thighs to maintain proper head placement and work those abs.

**POSITION 1:** Continue to inhale and switch legs, bringing your left knee to your chest while your left hand is on your left shin and your right hand is just below your knee, give your knee two hugs. Exhale to switch legs to bring your right knee to your chest, right hand on right shin and left hand on the knee; continue exhaling to switch legs to bring your left knee to your chest, left hand on shin and right hand on knee; this is one set. Exhale gradually to flatten your belly. Repeat 5 to 10 times.

## THE PAYOFF:

Gives you flat, sexy, strong abs.

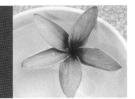

# Double Leg Stretch

REPLAY WEEKS ONE, TWO, FOUR

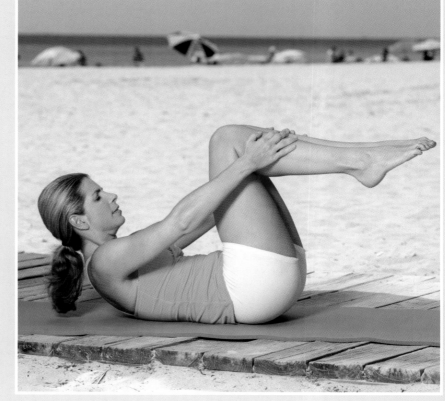

**STARTING POSITION:** Lie on your back with your knees to your chest and place your hands on your shins. Curl your chin to your chest and lift your head, neck, and upper back off the mat.

**TIPS AND TRICKS**

- Don't look at the ceiling; keep your chin to your chest and look between your thighs at all times. If you still feel tension, your abs might not be strong enough yet. Rest your head off the mat and move it from side to side between the two exercises.

- Don't bounce, jerk, or lift your lower back from the mat while your arms and legs move; your arms and legs are challenging your abs, so use them by scooping your belly button to your spine the whole time.

- Don't arch your back as your legs move away from your torso; keep your back flat against the mat the whole time. If you can't maintain a flat back, straighten your legs to the ceiling to reduce the stress on your lower back.

## THE PAYOFF:

Develops crazy-strong, flat abs.

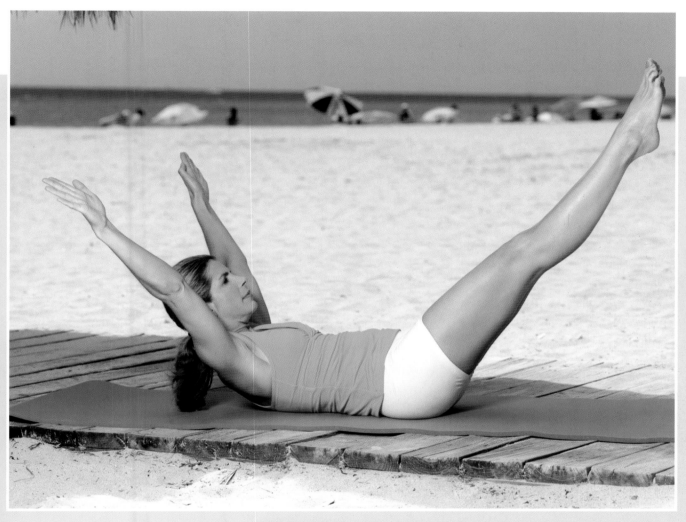

**POSITION 1:** In one motion, inhale to straighten your legs to the ceiling and reach your arms over your head, and begin to circle them behind you and around. Exhale to finish the circle, then use your abs to bring your knees to your chest. Give your knees a hug with your hands to empty your lungs of air—it's a lovely lower back stretch. Repeat 5 to 8 smooth flowing stretches.

# Straight Leg Scissors

REPLAY WEEK FOUR

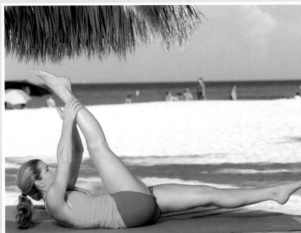

**STARTING POSITION:** Lie on your back with straight legs at a 90-degree angle. Lift your shoulders off the ground, and curl your chin to your chest. Drop your left leg to the floor so your toes are in line with your nose while holding your right ankle or calf. Inhale to stretch, then quickly pull your right leg to your forehead.

### TIPS AND TRICKS

- Don't strain your neck; your neck muscles may give out if you don't have the belly strength. Clasp your hands and place them behind your head for support while keeping your legs moving. If you still feel any strain, take a break.

- Don't bounce your torso; establish a continuous, smooth tempo, focusing on your breath. Also, if you don't have the hamstring flexibility, it may be difficult to straighten your legs, so bend your knees. Eventually, you'll get there!

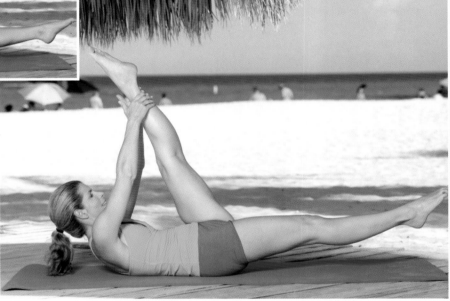

**POSITION 1:** Switch legs in a scissors-like motion, exhale, and stretch and pull the left leg, keeping your legs straight and flowing as the legs change position. Imagine scissoring your legs as if a piece of glass were between your legs, so you're holding your legs slightly apart.

## THE PAYOFF:

Uncovers lovely, flat abs.

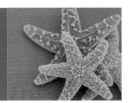

# Double Straight Leg Lift

## REPLAY WEEK FOUR

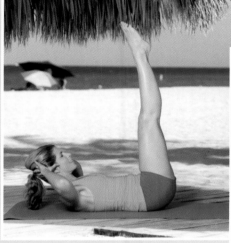

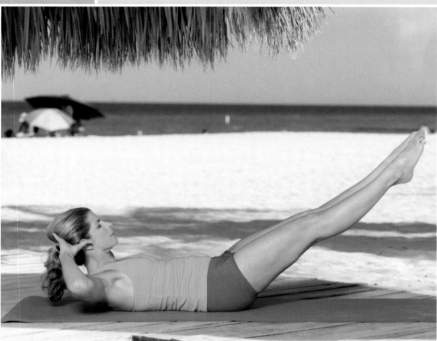

**STARTING POSITION:** Lie on your back with straight legs lengthening to the ceiling at a 90-degree angle. Clasp your hands behind your head for support, and open your shoulders. Scoop your belly button in and up, and be heavy in your torso.

### TIPS AND TRICKS

- Don't lift your lower back off the mat; only lower your legs without feeling this in your lower back. If you can't keep your back on the mat, bend your knees and dip your toes in the water. Don't strain your lower back.

- Don't forget to scoop, scoop, and scoop your abs.

**POSITION 1:** Inhale to lower your legs to the floor, only taking the legs as low as your back is anchored to the mat: no strain, no arch, no bulge! Exhale to lift your legs to a 90-degree angle, exhaling out every last breath to drop your belly button to your spine. Imagine a low seat belt is tightly fastened around your lower belly, from hip bone to hip bone, to feel your lower belly, or transverse muscles. Repeat 5 to 10 times.

## THE PAYOFF:

Takes you from so-so to stunning abs.

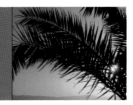

# Criss-Cross

REPLAY WEEK FOUR

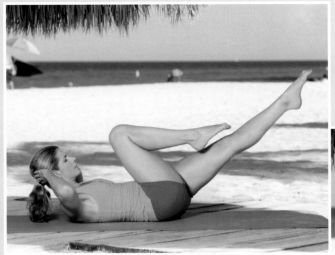

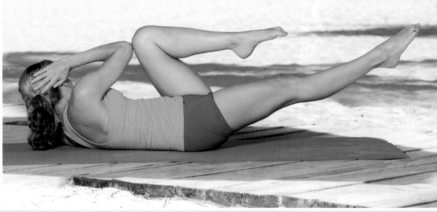

**STARTING POSITION:** Lie on your back with your knees bent at a 90-degree angle. Lift your shoulders off the ground, and curl your chin to your chest. Straighten your left leg so it's about nose level, toes in line with your nose, while your right knee nears your chest.

**TIPS AND TRICKS**

- Wring out your lungs with every exhale to get that yummy oblique work. Deepen your twist on every set; your elbow reaches past your knee while you look behind you. Slow down the tempo and hold the twist—it's killer!

**POSITION 1:** Inhale to twist your right elbow to left knee. Imagine your ribs collapsing or tightening around your belly. Repeat 5 to 10 times.

## THE PAYOFF:

Scorches your love handles.

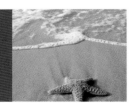

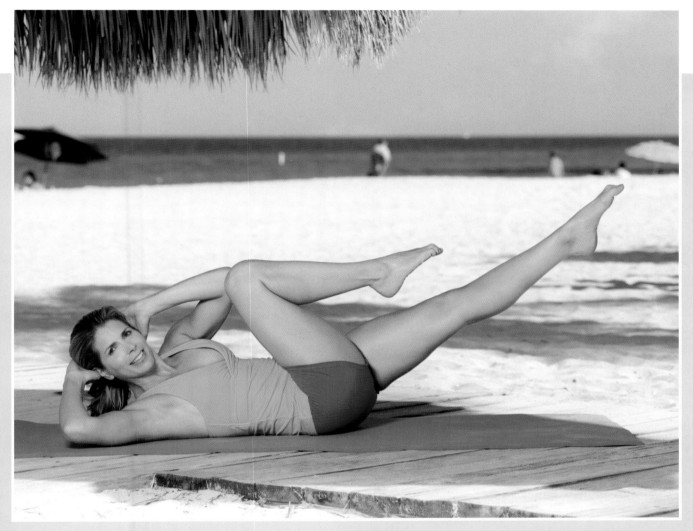

**POSITION 2:** Exhale to twist from your bottom rib so your torso moves your left elbow to your right knee, armpit to knee.

# Spine Stretch

REPLAY WEEKS ONE, TWO, FOUR, FIVE, SIX

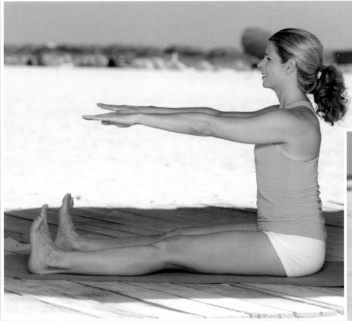

**STARTING POSITION:** Sit on your mat with your legs straight, a little wider than shoulder width apart, feet flexed. Lift your arms so they're parallel to your legs. Inhale to grow tall in your spine.

## TIPS AND TRICKS

- Don't move your lower body; turn on your hamstrings and flex your feet as you round over.
- Don't stretch forward; scoop your abs to stretch your spine and round over. You may feel a lovely hamstrings stretch, too.
- Don't slump in your lower back; sit on top of your butt bones, as though you're sitting on hot rocks.

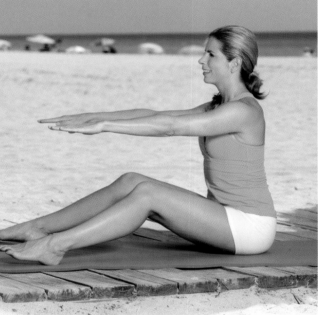

**MODIFIED POSITION:** If you have tight hamstrings and you're slumping in your lower back, modify the position by bending your knees or putting a small pad under your bottom.

## THE PAYOFF:

Develops a healthy, flexible spine.

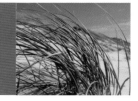

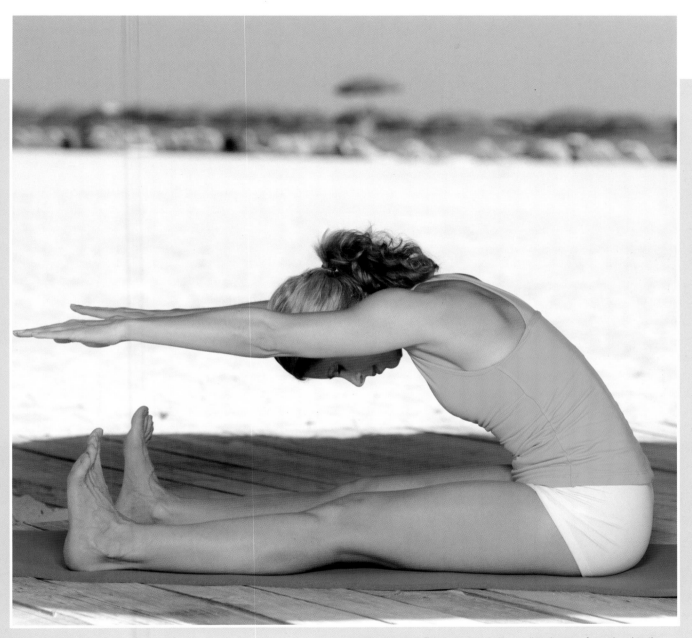

**POSITION 1:** Exhale to round over, curling the top of your head to the floor. Imagine a mean, ugly porcupine with long, sharp needles under your belly—scoop, scoop, scoop! As your fingertips stretch past your toes, scoop your abs to feel the stretch in your lower back. Inhale to roll up, vertebra on top of vertebra. Repeat 3 to 5 times.

# Open Leg Rocker

REPLAY WEEKS FOUR, FIVE, SIX

**STARTING POSITION:** Sit at the edge of the mat and slide your heels to your booty. Move your pubic bone to the ceiling and scoop your abs. Hold this scoop and then straighten your legs to make a "V." Your legs are a little wider than shoulder width apart. All limbs are straight, and your chin is on your chest.

**TIPS AND TRICKS**

- Stay active in your belly and you'll be able to balance better.

- Don't roll onto your neck; roll onto your upper back by scooping your abs. If you come up too quickly or flop to one side, slightly bend your knees and scoop. It's all about focus, balance, and control.

- Use your breath as you roll up; squeeze every ounce of air out to protect your lower back. Engage your pelvic floor to give you more power.

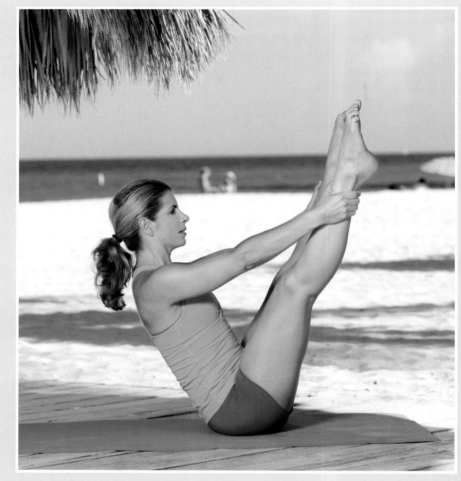

## THE PAYOFF:

A 100 percent belly strengthener that leads to flat, sexy abs.

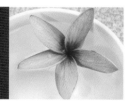

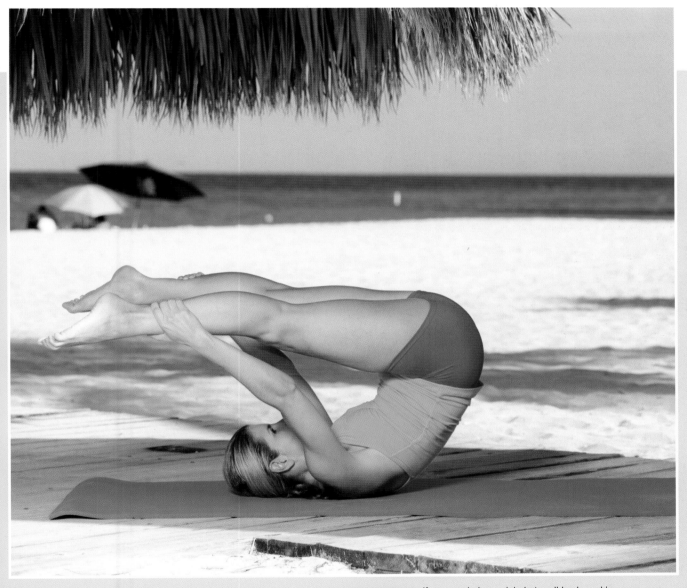

**POSITION 1:** If you can balance, inhale to roll back, making sure your weight lands on your shoulders and that the top of your head never touches the mat. Exhale to roll up, and scoop, scoop, and scoop to a balanced "V" position. Imagine a rocking chair; feel the rhythm of it rocking back and forth. Repeat 5 to 8 times.

# Corkscrew

REPLAY WEEKS ONE, TWO, FOUR, FIVE, SIX

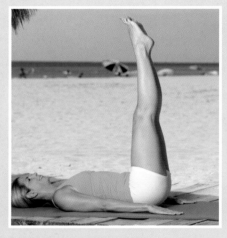

**STARTING POSITION:** Lie on your back with your legs straight at a 90-degree angle, feet in a Pilates "V." Straighten your arms by your sides, lengthening your fingertips. Slide your shoulder blades down your back.

**TIPS AND TRICKS**

- Don't lift your head or shoulders off the mat; keep your circles small so you can maintain good form until you get stronger.

- Don't separate your legs; squeeze your inner thighs to give you lots of power!

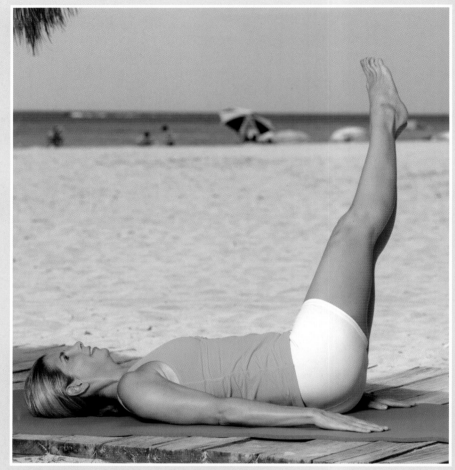

**POSITION 1:** Make a small circle with your legs to the left, letting the right hip come off the mat slightly. Keep your knees and ankles together the entire time.

## THE PAYOFF:

Scorches those love handles.

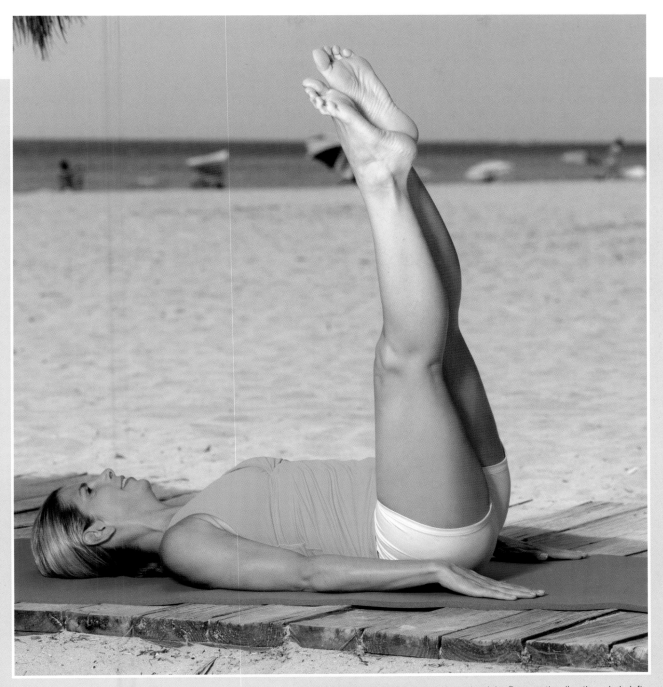

**POSITION 2:** Complete the circle to the right. Reverse the direction, circle left and finish right; that's one complete set. Imagine a string pulling your toes to the ceiling, so lengthen your legs away from your hips, keeping your knees and ankles together. Do 3 to 5 circles.

# Saw

REPLAY WEEKS ONE, TWO, FOUR

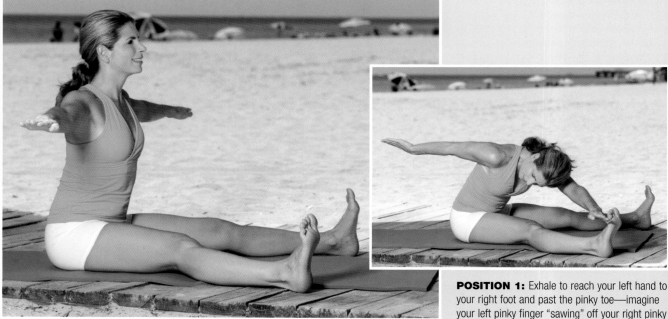

**STARTING POSITION:** Sit tall on the mat with your legs straight and a little wider than shoulder width apart, feet flexed. Lift your arms out to the sides of your body, and reach your fingertips long, palms down. Inhale to grow tall in your spine, lifting your ribs slightly up off your pelvis to initiate the twist.

### TIPS AND TRICKS

- Don't bounce as you twist; it's a lengthening from your waist as you reach your arms farther apart.
- Don't do any rotation if you have a back injury; please ask your doctor if "rotation" or "twisting" is appropriate for you.
- Don't slump in your lower back; sit on top of your butt bones like you're sitting on hot rocks!

**POSITION 1:** Exhale to reach your left hand to your right foot and past the pinky toe—imagine your left pinky finger "sawing" off your right pinky toe while your left ear moves closer to your right knee; pulse for 3 counts while stretching your right hand behind you, palm up. With each pulse, twist a little farther, exhaling every ounce of air from your lungs as if you were wringing out a dirty dish towel. Inhale to return to the starting position even taller in your spine.

## THE PAYOFF:

Leads to a stunning waist and strong obliques.

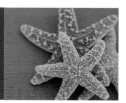

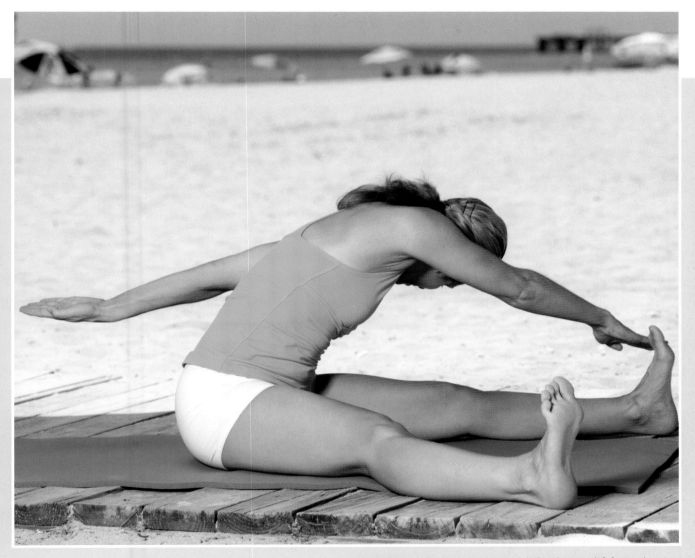

**POSITION 2:** Exhale to reach your right hand to your left foot and past the pinky toe. Imagine sawing off your pinky toe while your right ear moves closer to your left knee; pulse for 3 counts while stretching your left hand behind you, palm up. With each pulse, twist a little farther, exhaling every ounce of air out of your lungs. Inhale to return to the starting position even taller in your spine. Repeat 3 to 5 times.

# Swan

REPLAY WEEKS ONE, TWO, FOUR, FIVE, SIX

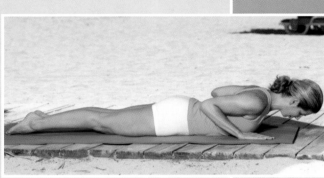

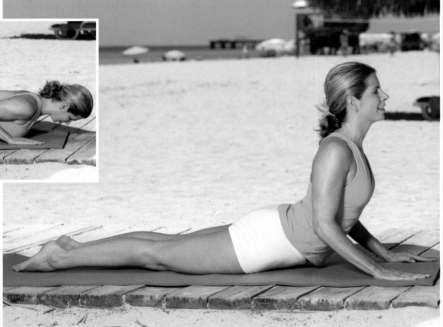

**STARTING POSITION:** Lie on your stomach with your legs straight, placing your hands directly under your shoulders, palms down. Elbows are close to your rib cage. Put some action in your butt cheeks and lift your belly button toward your spine.

**TIPS AND TRICKS**

- Don't forget about the principles of extension: hip bones and pubic bone press into the mat; booty and hamstrings are engaged; armpits are dropped to your hips.

- Don't move your elbows to the sides of your chest; imagine a pencil between your arms and your rib cage, then squeeze it and shave your elbows past your rib cage to keep your elbows close to your body.

- Don't elevate your shoulders as you rock up and down; lower your shoulder blades down your back to stabilize your shoulders and open your chest.

**POSITION 1:** Inhale and slowly lift your chest off the mat, leading with your breastbone. Lift as high as you can, without feeling any pressure in your lower back. Exhale, lower to the mat, and quickly inhale up so you're rocking on your belly. Repeat 3 to 5 times.

## THE PAYOFF:

Gives you a healthy belly and strong, fit back.

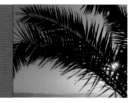

# Single Leg Kick

REPLAY WEEKS ONE, TWO, FOUR, FIVE, SIX

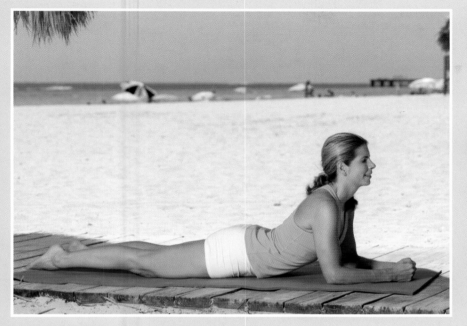

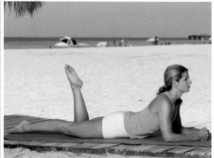

**POSITION 1:** Inhale, kick your right heel to your butt and then kick again.

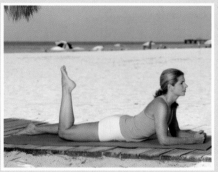

**POSITION 2:** Exhale, kick your right heel to your butt, and then kick again. Keep a steady rhythm going, both legs should be moving at the same time. Repeat 5 to 8 times.

**STARTING POSITION:** Lie on your stomach and lift your belly button toward your spine. Firm up your fanny and press your hip bones and pubic bone into the mat. Put your elbows directly under your shoulders and toward the belly to make an upside down "V," and press your elbows into the mat. Make two fists, and place your knuckles together.

### TIPS AND TRICKS

- Don't jiggle your booty; keep your pelvis stable and firm up your fanny.
- Don't round your shoulders; lift your head out of your shoulders as your breastbone lifts to the ceiling.
- Don't sag your belly; stay active to support your lower back. If you feel any lower back strain, put a pillow underneath your pelvis.

## THE PAYOFF:

Firms up your backside.

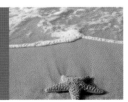

# Double Leg Kick

REPLAY WEEKS ONE, TWO, FOUR, FIVE, SIX

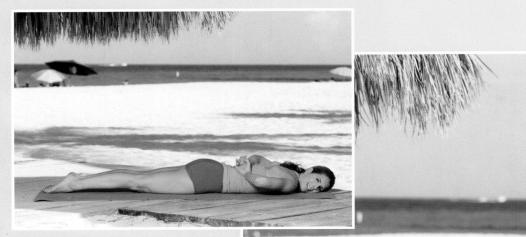

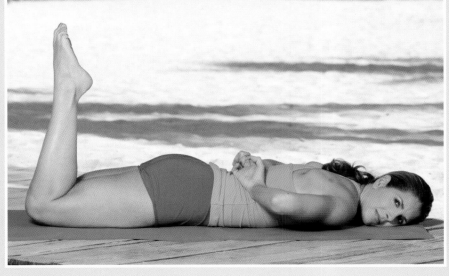

**STARTING POSITION:** Lie on your stomach with your legs straight, left cheek on the mat. Clasp your left hand around two fingers on your right hand, and position them in the middle of your back, elbows to the floor. You should feel a nice stretch across your back.

**TIPS AND TRICKS**

- Don't forget the principles of extension: press your hip bones and pubic bone into the mat; firm up your fanny and hamstrings; and don't flab your belly.

- Don't worry about the hand placement; just rest your hands on your lower back, palms up. When you lift into extension, just straighten your arms by your sides, palms down.

**POSITION 1:** Inhale to cue your body, then exhale to draw your heels to your bum; pulse three times to work your hamstrings. Don't lift your hip bones off the mat.

## THE PAYOFF:

Gives you a simply gorgeous, fit back.

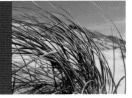

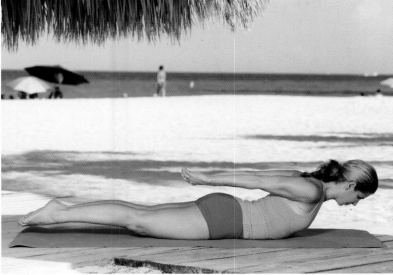

**POSITION 2:** Inhale into an extension of your spine while moving your arms down your back to lift your chest off the mat. The shoulder blades pull together to roll the shoulders back as you lift your clasped hands toward the ceiling to stretch your chest. Imagine shaving your arms down your back to draw your shoulders down.

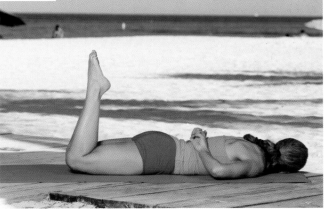

**POSITION 3:** Turn your cheek to the right, then exhale to draw your heels to your bum; pulse three times to work your hamstrings. Don't lift your hip bones off the mat. Do 3 to 5 reps, counting the right and left cheek as one rep.

# Neck Pull

REPLAY WEEK FOUR

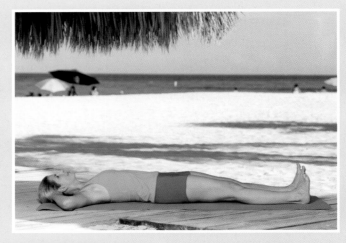

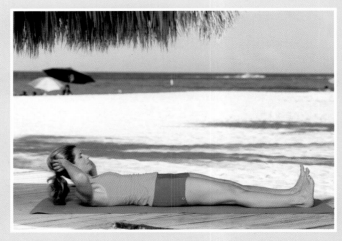

**STARTING POSITION:** Lie on your back with your legs straight, feet parallel and hip width apart. Clasp your hands and place them behind your head so you can see your elbows out to the sides. Press your heels away from your hips, and be heavy in your heinie. Drop the backs of your shoulders against the mat, and slide your shoulder blades down your back.

**TIPS AND TRICKS**

- Don't hide your face as you roll up; your elbows are in your peripheral vision or lengthened out to the sides.
- Don't plop down; as you roll down, press your heels away from your hips, and scoop!
- Don't strain your lower back; if you feel a twinge in your lower back, bend your knees and follow the steps above.

**POSITION 1:** Inhale to lift your head off the mat and curl your chin to your chest to initiate peeling your spine off the mat, keep your neck long.

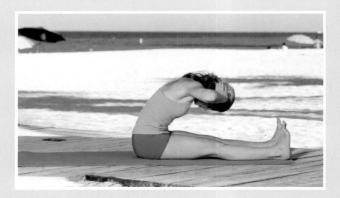

**POSITION 2:** Exhale to round over, bringing your nose to your belly button.

## THE PAYOFF:

Builds sexy, strong, and flat abs.

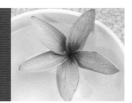

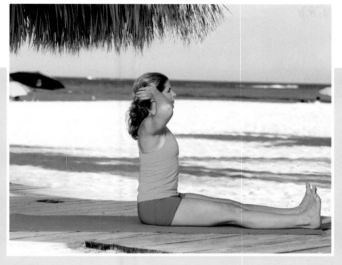

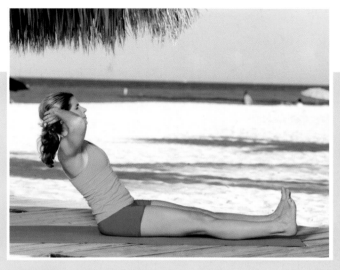

**POSITION 3:** Inhale to stack your vertebrae as you uncurl your spine, lifting your head to the ceiling until you're sitting out of your hips.

**POSITION 4:** Still inhaling, lean back so your stomach is flat, heels pressing away from your hips. Imagine sitting on hot rocks to lift from your butt cheeks as your torso turns into a piece of glass.

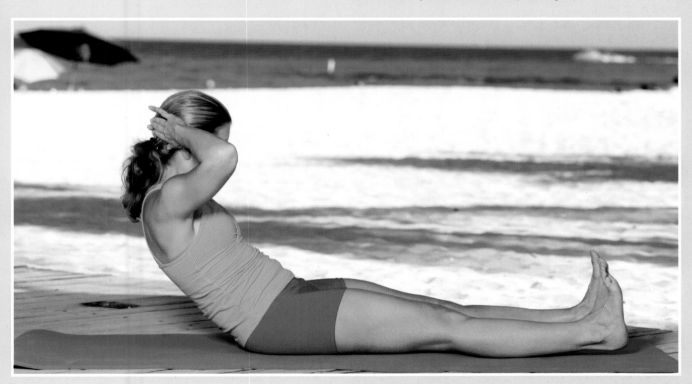

**POSITION 5:** Exhale to scoop your abs, moving your pubic bone to the ceiling, and roll down vertebra by vertebra. Repeat 3 to 5 times.

# Shoulder Bridge with One Leg

REPLAY WEEK FOUR

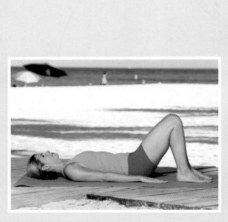

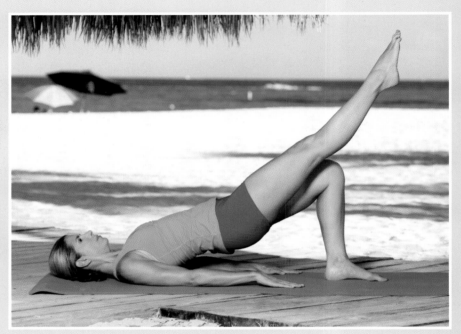

**STARTING POSITION:** Lie on your back with your arms straight by your sides and place your feet about hip width apart. Inhale to cue your body.

## TIPS AND TRICKS

- Don't sag in your booty; keep your hips even and maintain a neutral position to build your core strength.
- Use your abs; stay solid from your breastbone to your pubic bone even as you lift your leg, the tendency is for one hip to droop.

**POSITION 1:** Exhale to scoop your abs and lift your spine off the mat vertebra by vertebra. Once you're stabilized, lift your right leg and count to 5 to challenge your core even more! Inhale to roll down, vertebra by vertebra.

## THE PAYOFF:

Perks up your booty and creates a strong core.

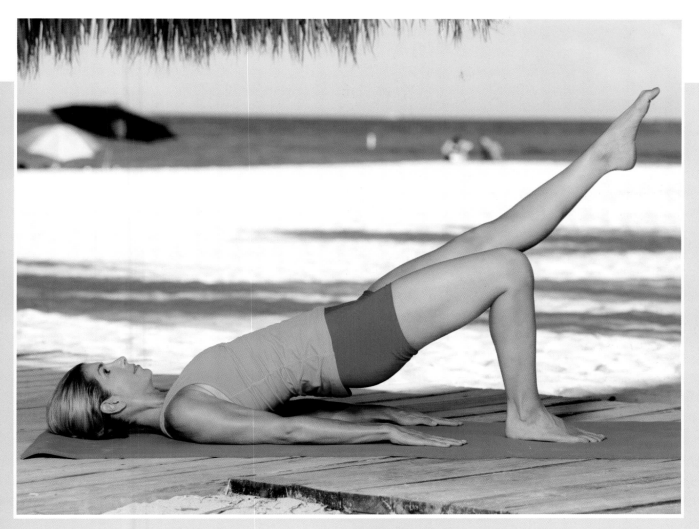

**POSITION 2:** Exhale to scoop your abs and lift your spine off the mat vertebra by vertebra. Lift your left leg and count to 5 to challenge your core even more! Inhale to roll down, vertebra by vertebra, as if you were lying in sand. Imagine a sling is hanging from the ceiling to hoist your hips and prevent your bottom from sinking into the mat. Repeat 3 to 5 times.

# Teaser 2

REPLAY WEEK FOUR

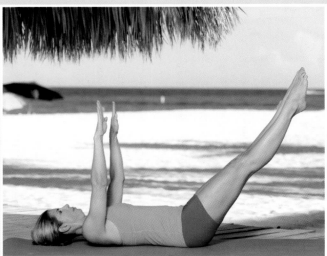

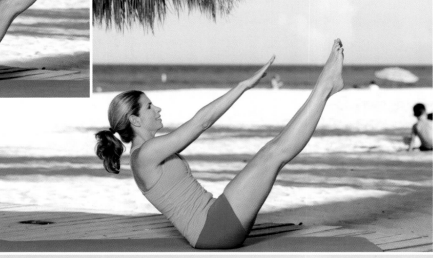

**STARTING POSITION:** Lie on your back with your legs straight so your toes are in line with your nose, place your feet in a Pilates "V," and straighten your arms over your head.

**TIPS AND TRICKS**

- Don't strain in your lower back; if you're not ready for the Teaser 2, turn back to week one (p. 56) and do the Teaser 1.
- Don't plop down; scoop and lower with control.

**POSITION 1:** Inhale to lift your arms to your legs at the same time, coming into a "V," fingertips lifting to your toes. Scoop, scoop, scoop to work your abs and protect your back. Exhale to roll down slowly to the mat. Repeat 3 to 5 times.

## THE PAYOFF:

Uncovers the sexiest, sleekest abs and that's a promise.

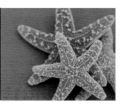

# The Seal

REPLAY WEEKS ONE, TWO, FOUR, FIVE, SIX

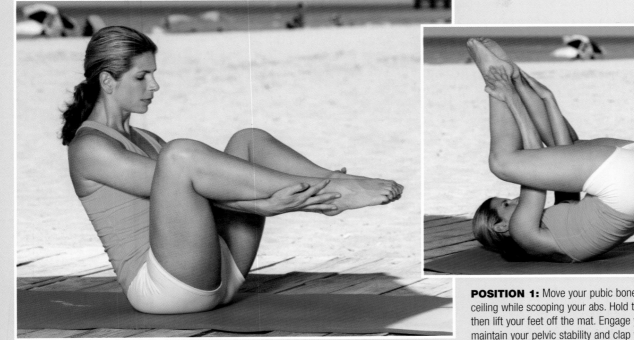

**STARTING POSITION:** Sit at the edge of the mat and slide your heels to your booty. Drive into your legs and wrap your arms under and around so your hands end up on the outside of your ankles. Look at your belly as you drop your chin to your chest, rounding your spine.

## TIPS AND TRICKS

- Engage your inner thighs when you clap your heels.
- Don't roll onto your head or neck; it's the upper back and shoulders that absorb the weight of your body.

**POSITION 1:** Move your pubic bone to the ceiling while scooping your abs. Hold this scoop, then lift your feet off the mat. Engage your abs to maintain your pelvic stability and clap your heels and bark like a seal. (Why not? It's free and fun.) Inhale to roll back to your upper back, only. Exhale to roll up. Pause, clap your heels 3 times, and roll again, scooping your belly the whole time to find your balance. Repeat 8 to 10 times.

## THE PAYOFF:

Leads to a flexible, fit spine.

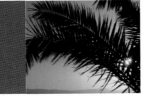

# SUNDAY: TAKING IT EASY–YOU'RE WORTH IT!

Take today off, knowing you'll soon have a killer figure. Keep up the great work by adding some healthy eating habits that will get you bikini ready:

- **Munch on nuts:** Nuts, especially almonds, are heart healthy. According to the journal *Obesity*, munching them regularly may cut your risk of gaining weight by 30 percent over two years.

- **Get more bananas:** Nature's perfect food is chock-full of mood-lifting vitamin B and can give you enough energy for a 90-minute workout. Add some almond butter, and you have perfect combo for a fit body!

- **Ditch the soft drinks:** Soft drinks, even diet ones are horrible for your bikini belly, and there are studies to prove it. Instead, add more antioxidant-rich teas: black, red, white, and green to boost your precious nutrients and lose inches around the bikini middle.

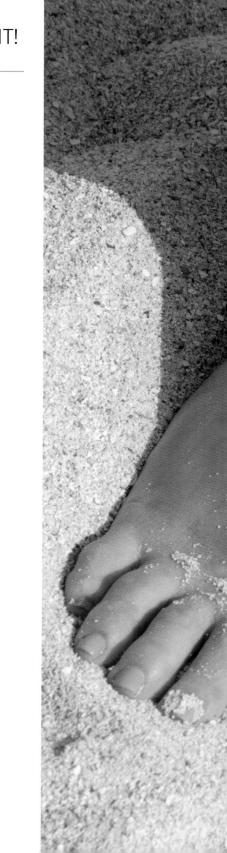

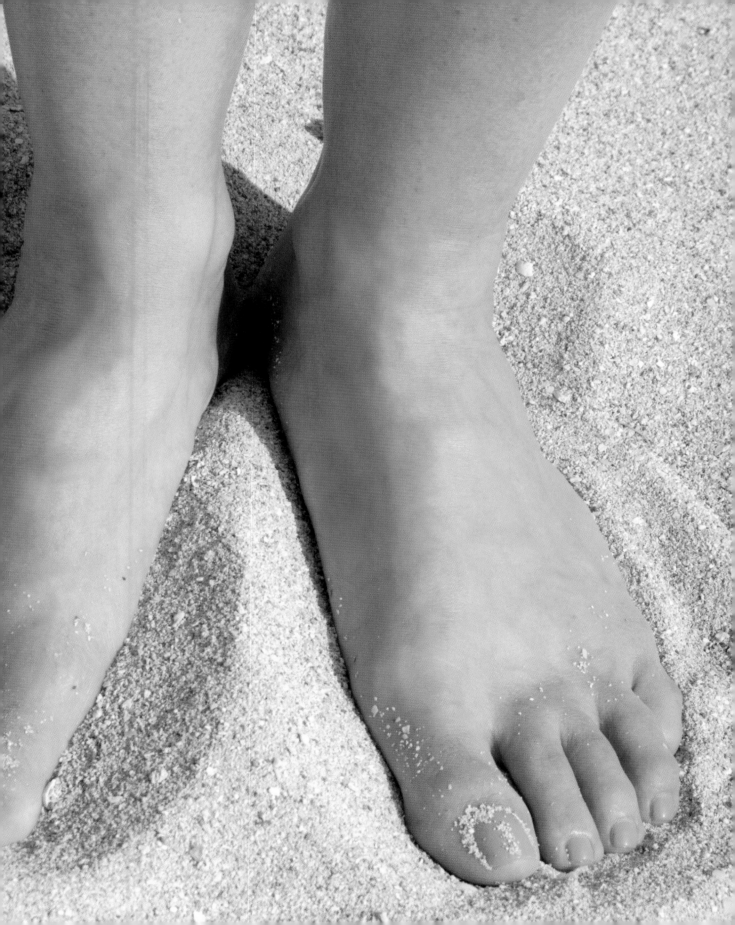

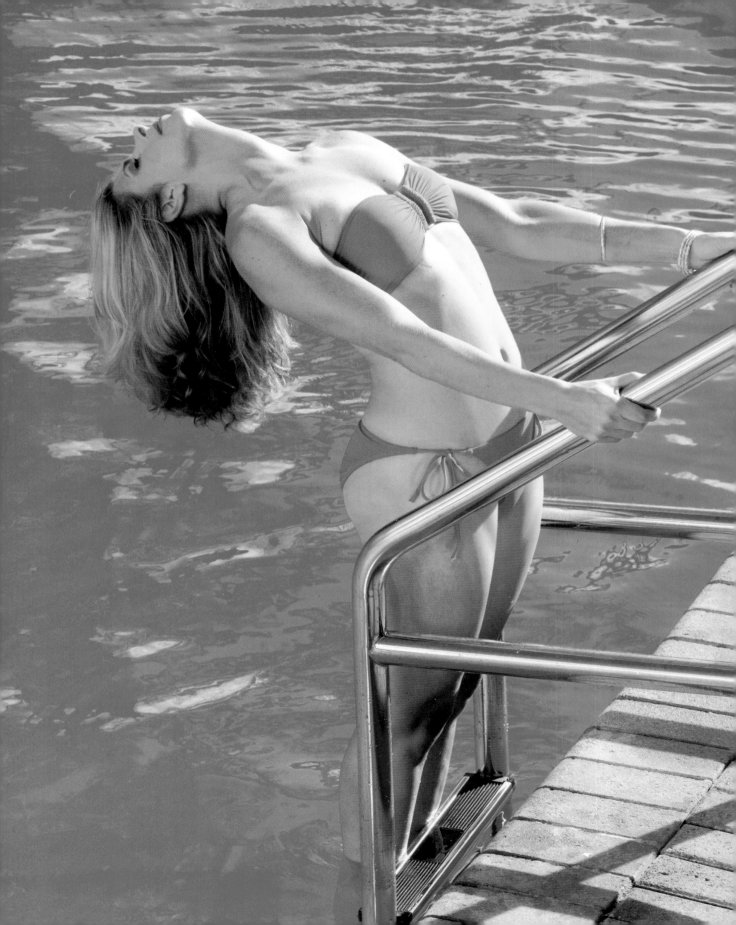

# week four

## INNER BEAUTY ... OUTER BOOTY

If venturing out to the beach baring it all has got you all twisted inside, then RELAX. This week, you'll shed your bikini anxiety and boost your bikini confidence with toning exercises that will perk up your bum and flatten your tum. You'll no longer be the girl sitting next to the girl in a bikini—and that's a promise.

| | |
|---|---|
| **MONDAY** | Burning It Off with Boot-Camp-Strength Intervals |
| **TUESDAY** | Stepping on It with Steady-State Cardio |
| **WEDNESDAY** | Lifting Your Bottom Line with Pilates |
| **THURSDAY** | Burning It Off with Boot-Camp-Strength Intervals |
| **FRIDAY** | Stepping on It with Steady-State Cardio |
| **SATURDAY** | Lifting Your Bottom Line with Pilates |
| **SUNDAY** | Enjoying Yourself! |

# week four

M T W T

| MONDAY | TUESDAY | WEDNESDAY | THURSDAY |
|---|---|---|---|
| Burning It Off with Boot-Camp-Strength Intervals | Stepping on It with Steady-State Cardio | Lifting Your Bottom Line with Pilates | Burning It Off with Boot-Camp-Strength Intervals |
| **Set 1**<br><br>Speedy Legs with Hands<br><br>Front Plank<br><br>Overhead Triceps Extension | **1**. 3 minutes: Warm up at moderate pace at intensity level 5<br><br>**2**. 50 minutes: Step it up and be breathless and sweaty with intensity level 6 to 8<br><br>**3**. 2 minutes: Cool down at an intensity level of 3 to 4 | **After doing the Pilates Abs in week three, do these Pilates exercises today:**<br><br>Standing Sweep Kick<br><br>Standing<br>  Beat … Beat … UP<br><br>Standing Side Passé<br><br>Standing Leg Circle (front and back)<br><br>Standing Outer Thigh Lift<br><br>Standing Booty Lift<br><br>Standing Front Kick<br><br>Standing Bicycle<br><br>Standing Curtsy | **Set 1**<br><br>Speedy Legs with Hands<br><br>Front Plank<br><br>Overhead Triceps Extension |
| **Set 2**<br><br>Hop Squat<br><br>Right- and Left-Side Plank | | | **Set 2**<br><br>Hop Squat<br><br>Right- and Left-Side Plank |
| **Set 3**<br><br>Plank with Jumps on Step<br><br>Plank with Outer Thigh Lift<br><br>Push-ups | | | **Set 3**<br><br>Plank with Jumps on Step<br><br>Plank with Outer Thigh Lift<br><br>Push-ups |

|   | **FRIDAY** | **SATURDAY** | **SUNDAY** |
|---|---|---|---|

## FRIDAY

### Stepping on It with Steady-State Cardio

1. 3 minutes: Warm up at moderate pace at intensity level 5
2. 50 minutes: Step it up and be breathless and sweaty with intensity level 6 to 8
3. 2 minutes: Cool down at an intensity level of 3 to 4

## SATURDAY

### Lifting Your Bottom Line with Pilates

**After doing the Pilates Abs in week three, do these Pilates exercises today:**

Standing Sweep Kick

Standing
   Beat … Beat … UP

Standing Side Passé

Standing Leg Circle (front and back)

Standing Outer Thigh Lift

Standing Booty Lift

Standing Front Kick

Standing Bicycle

Standing Curtsy

## SUNDAY

### Enjoying Yourself!

OFF

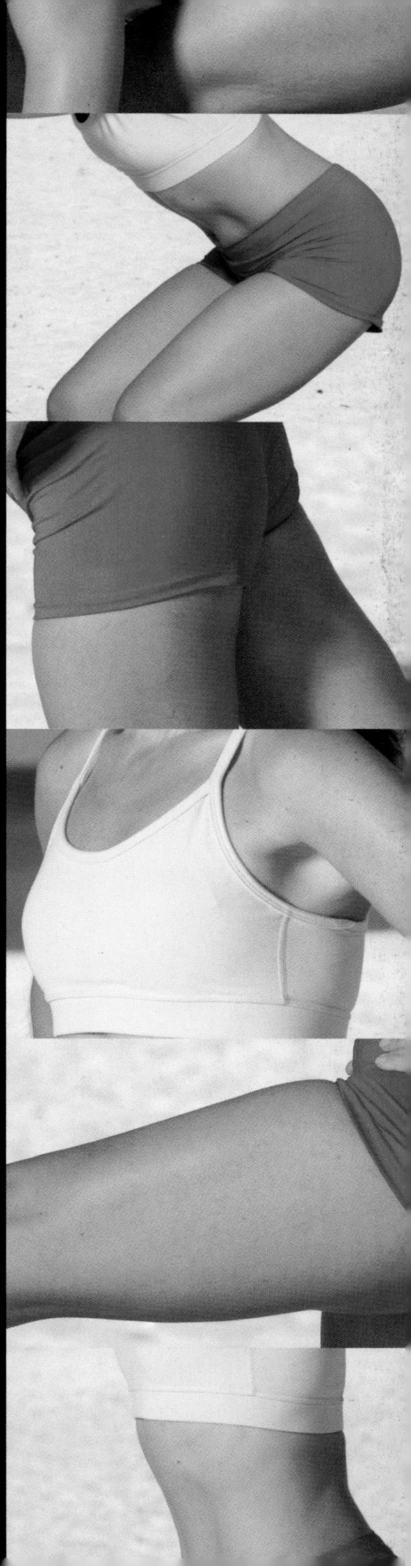

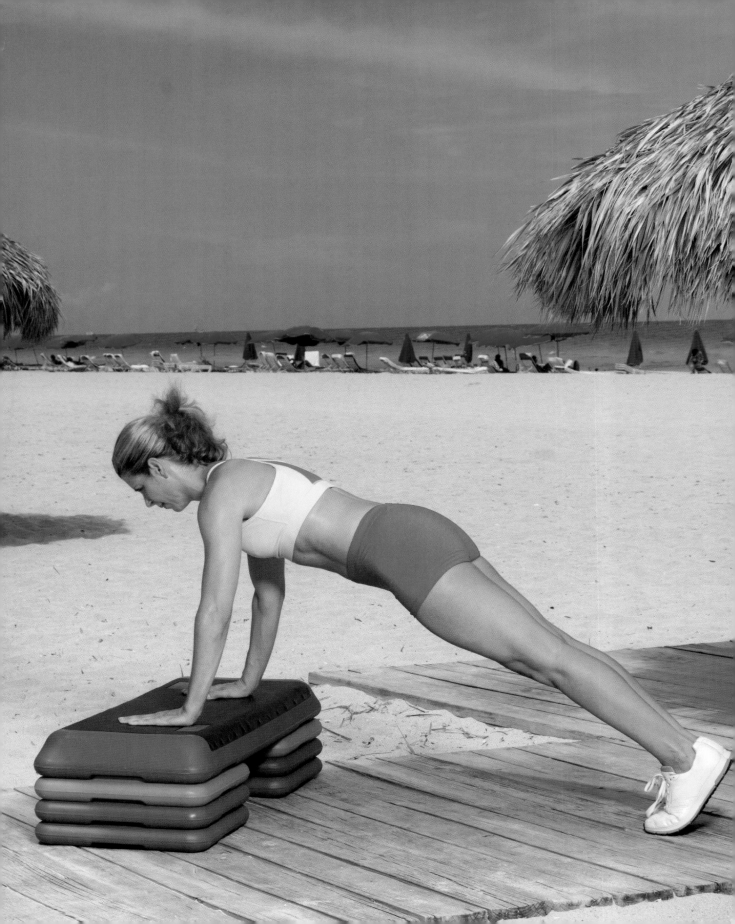

# MONDAY: BURNING IT OFF
## WITH BOOT-CAMP-STRENGTH INTERVALS

It's pretty simple, your best bikini body means calories in versus calories out. To define your muscles, you need to keep the fat burn revving, and that means working multiple muscles at once. Because you're already feeling stronger (thanks, core), these exercises take it up to a jump-off-the-jiggle level. Don't forget, this boot camp workout includes cardio, core, and strength training. You'll do a series of intense moves to keep your heart rate up while moving from exercise to exercise with no more than 30 seconds of rest, alternating between heavy breathing and a not-overly-demanding recovery interval. You'll need a couple sets of dumbbells: 15 to 20 pounds (7 to 9 kg) for your legs and 8 to 10 pounds (4 to 5 kg) for your arms.

To do this boot camp workout you'll do Set 1 three times, doing 15 to 20 reps of each exercise in that set, and then repeat the entire set two more times. For example, complete 15 to 20 slow and controlled reps of each exercise unless I tell you differently: Speedy Legs with Hands, Front Plank (hold for 30 to 60 seconds), and Overhead Triceps Extension. Repeat that set two times before moving on to Set 2, and then finish with Set 3. Total time should be about 45 minutes to 1 hour. If you're not clear on what a set or a rep is, flip to the introduction of this book. And don't forget to warm up on the treadmill for 5 minutes at 3.5 mph (5.5 kph).

**SET 1**

Speedy Legs with Hands

Front Plank

Overhead Triceps Extension

**SET 2**

Hop Squat

Right- and Left-Side Plank

**SET 3**

Plank with Jumps on Step

Plank with Outer Thigh Lift

Push-ups

# Speedy Legs with Hands

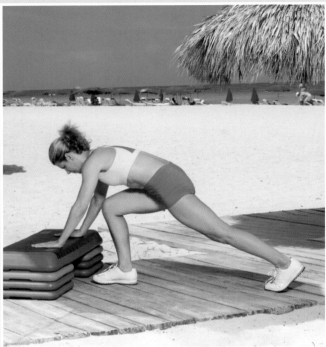

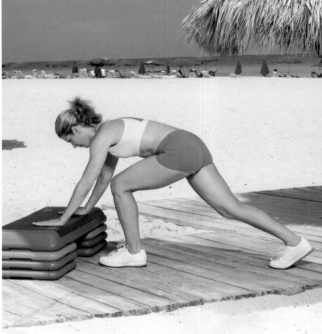

**STARTING POSITION:** Place your hands on the bench and get into a deep lunge position. Look down.

**TIPS AND TRICKS**

- Don't lean forward; your torso will naturally come forward slightly as you squat. If you want extra butt work, sit back in your heels so your hips and knees are parallel to the floor.

- Don't forget to engage your abs to support your lower back.

**POSITION 1:** As quickly as you can, alternate your legs from left to right in the lunge position. Repeat 20 times.

## THE PAYOFF:

Shrinks legs, butt, and core.

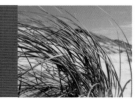

# Front Plank

REPLAY WEEK THREE

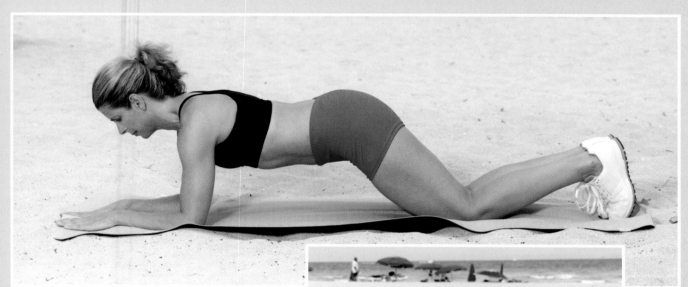

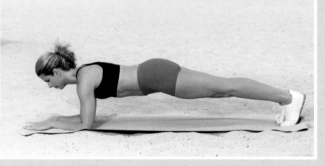

**STARTING POSITION:** On your knees, place your elbows directly under your shoulders, palms down. With your toes curled under, place your heels together.

## TIPS AND TRICKS

- Don't sag your belly; gently lift your belly button toward your spine to strengthen your core while giving your lower back support.
- Don't forget to firm up your fanny, inner thighs, and pelvic floor; oh-so-much power is wasted if you don't use them!
- Don't elevate your shoulders; draw your shoulder blades down your back to engage your upper back.
- Don't drop your head; gaze at the floor as you lengthen from the top of your head.

**POSITION 1:** Lift your legs, pelvis, and torso off the floor in one motion. Balance on your toes and elbows, keeping your back perfectly straight; imagine that everything from your head to your heels is like steel. Hold for 30 to 60 seconds, and then do 2 more reps.

# THE PAYOFF:

Sculpts all over and strengthens your core.

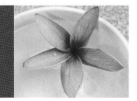

# Overhead Triceps Extension

REPLAY WEEK THREE

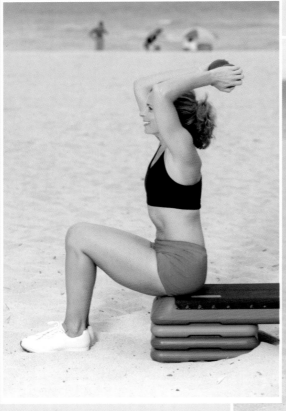

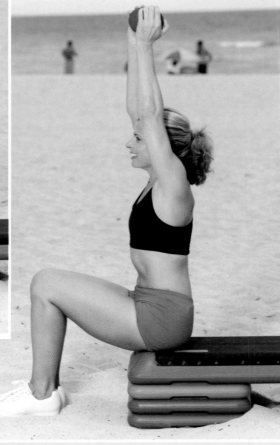

**STARTING POSITION:** Sit on a bench or stand and hold an 8- to 10-pound (4 to 5 kg) dumbbell in your hands. Lift your arms over your head and bend your arms so the dumbbell is behind your head, keeping your shoulders down.

### TIPS AND TRICKS

- Don't round your spine; keep your abs active and lengthen from the top of your head.
- Don't let your shoulders lift toward your ears; try to relax your upper back.

**POSITION 1:** Straighten your arms to the ceiling, leading with your knuckles. Keep your upper arms still so you can fully extend your arms. Do 15 to 20 reps.

## THE PAYOFF:

Lets you say good-bye to flabby arms.

# Hop Squat

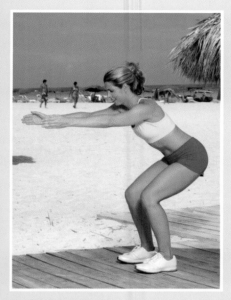

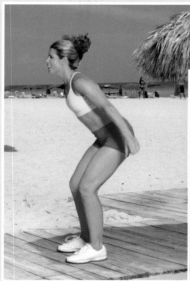

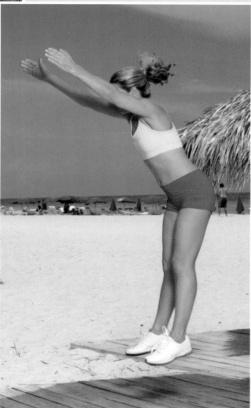

**STARTING POSITION:** Sit in a squat position with your thighs parallel to the floor and your knees aligned with your second and third toes. Straighten your arms out in front of you. Look forward or slightly up.

### TIPS AND TRICKS

- Don't lean forward; your torso will naturally come forward slightly as you squat. If you want extra butt work, sit back in your heels so your hips and knees are parallel to the floor.

- Don't turn your knees in; keep your knees stable and your toes facing forward as you squat.

- Don't forget your sexy posture; your torso is straight and your shoulders are relaxed.

- Don't arch your lower back; engage your abs to support your lower back.

**POSITION 1:** Keep your chest lifted and your spine straight as you begin to jump.

**POSITION 2:** Explode up, then out in front, landing in a squat; continue jumping for about 15 steps. Imagine a bunny hop!

## THE PAYOFF:

Reduces the jiggle in your abs, butt, and legs.

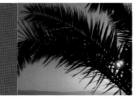

# Right- and Left-Side Plank

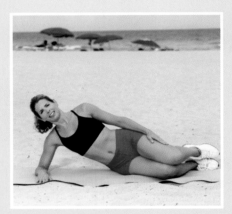

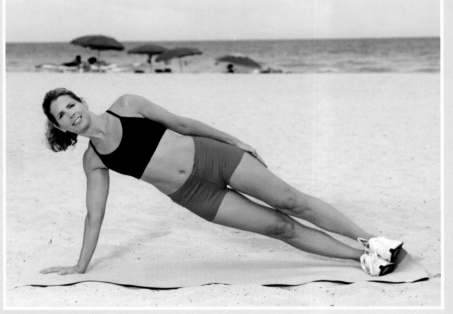

**STARTING POSITION:** Sit on your right side with your knees slightly pulled into your body, stacking your knees on top of one another. Place your hand on the floor slightly away your shoulder.

**POSITION 1:** Lift your torso, hips, and legs off the floor in one motion. Balance on your right hand and on the right leading edge of your foot, stacking your feet on top of one another.

## TIPS AND TRICKS

- Don't droop your torso in the middle; focus on your breath work and lift your trunk to the ceiling.
- Don't hang in your wrist; your wrist should line up under your shoulder and lift, lift, lift!
- If you can't maintain good form, do this plank on your elbows as shown in position 1 of Plank with Outer Thigh Lift (pp. 114 and 168).

## THE PAYOFF:

Takes inches off your waist and uncovers your sexy abs.

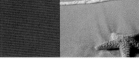

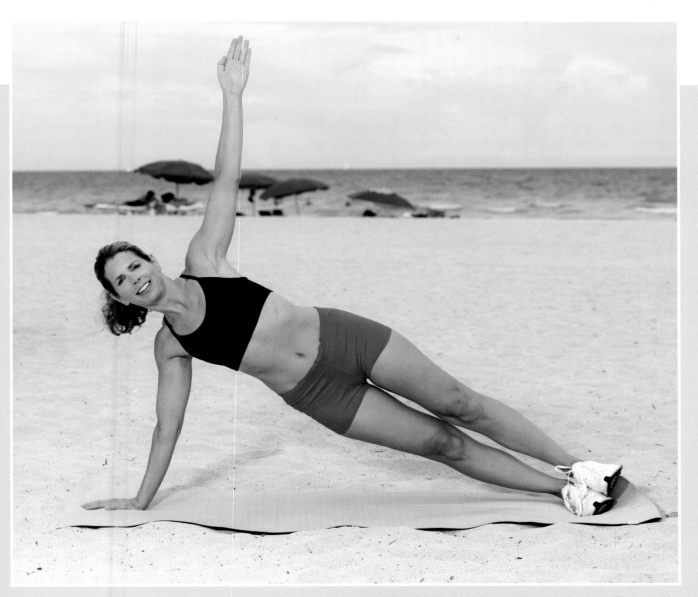

**POSITION 2:** Lift your left arm to the ceiling, forming a "T" shape with your body. Repeat 3 times, holding for 15 seconds, and then switch sides.

# Plank with Jumps on Step

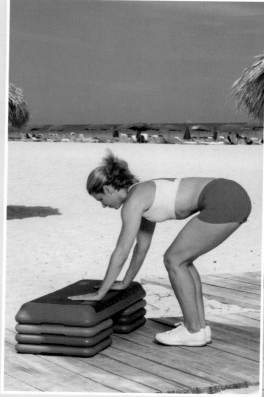

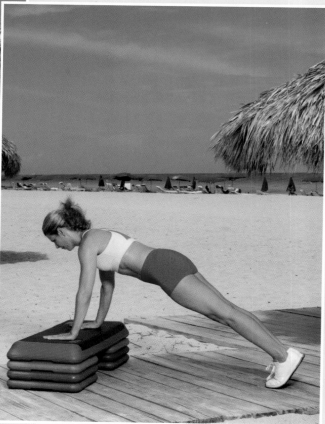

**STARTING POSITION:** Place your hands on a step, palms down, making sure your elbows are directly underneath your shoulders. Stand behind the step.

### TIPS AND TRICKS

- Don't sag in your lower back as you jump into plank position; lift your belly button toward your spine to support your lower back.

- Don't drop your head; look at the floor or keep your head in line with your spine.

**POSITION 1:** In one motion, jump back into a plank position, keeping your back perfectly straight; imagine that everything from your head to your heels is hard like steel.

## THE PAYOFF:

Leads to allover shrinkage and a mega sexy core.

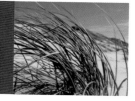

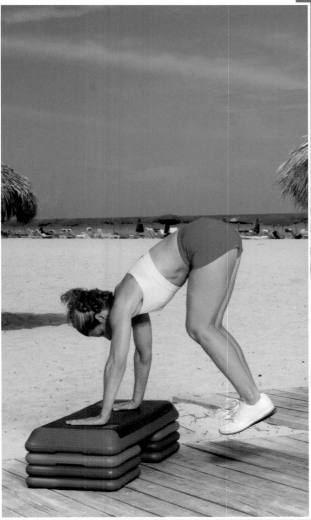

**POSITION 2:** Jump in toward the step.

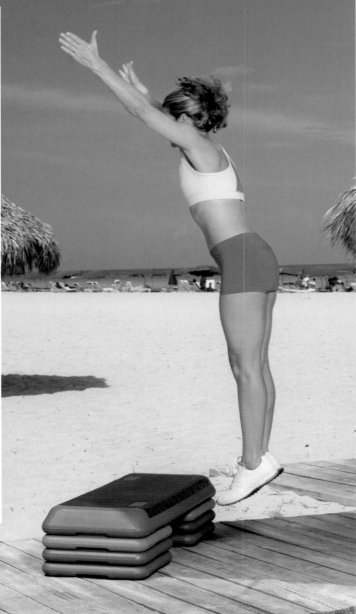

**POSITION 3:** Jump (explode) to the ceiling, using your arms to lift you even higher and then jump back to plank. Repeat for 15 to 20 reps.

# Plank with Outer Thigh Lift

REPLAY WEEK THREE

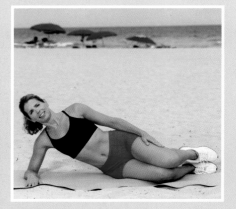

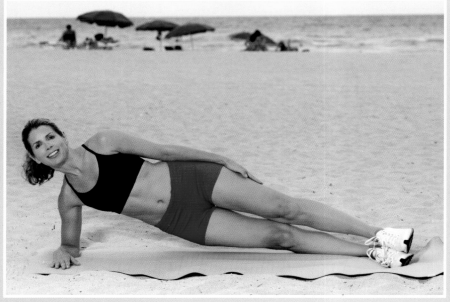

**STARTING POSITION:** Sit on your right side with your knees slightly pulled into your body, stacking your knees on top of one another. Place your elbow on the floor slightly out from your shoulder, fingertips away from your torso.

**TIPS AND TRICKS**

- Don't droop your torso; focus on your breath work and lift your torso to the ceiling.

- Don't hang in your neck or shoulders as you lift your leg. Just don't lower and lift, hold the leg up until you have enough strength to maintain good form.

**POSITION 1:** Lift your torso, hips, and legs off the floor in one motion. Balance on your right elbow and on the right leading edge of your foot, stacking your feet on top of one another.

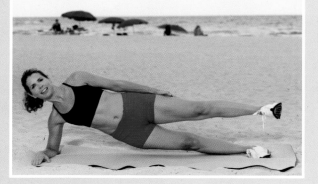

**POSITION 2:** Lift your top leg up toward the ceiling and then lower it to the plank (bottom leg). Repeat 5 to 8 times, and then switch sides.

## THE PAYOFF:

Sculpts all over and de-dimples your thighs.

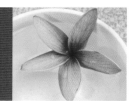

# Push-ups

REPLAY WEEK THREE

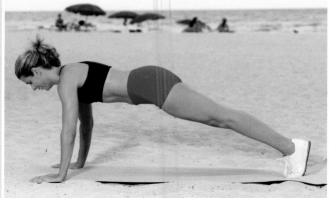

**STARTING POSITION:** On your knees, place your hands on the floor directly under your shoulders, palms down. With your toes curled under, place your heels together and lift your legs, pelvis, and torso off the floor in one motion. Balance on your toes and elbows, keeping your back perfectly straight, imagining that everything from your head to your heels is like steel.

## TIPS AND TRICKS

- Don't sag your belly; gently lift your belly button toward your spine to strengthen your core while giving your lower back support.

- Don't forget to firm up your fanny, inner thighs, and pelvic floor; oh-so-much power is wasted if you don't use them!

- Don't elevate your shoulders; draw your shoulder blades down your back to engage your upper back, and don't lower your torso as much.

- Don't drop your head; look at the floor as you lengthen from the top of your head.

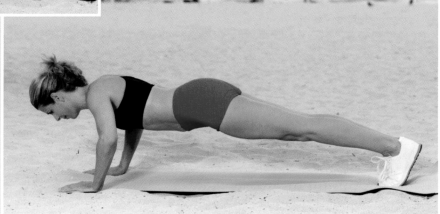

**POSITION 1:** Bend your elbows at the sides to lower your body to the floor. Push up to starting position. Do 15 to 20 reps.

## THE PAYOFF:

Sculpts all over and develops a beautiful chest.

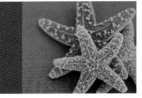

# TUESDAY: STEPPING ON IT WITH STEADY-STATE CARDIO

This week you're climbing your way to a leaner you! That's right, get jiggy with the stair stepper, and it will do amazing things for your butt and legs. Do a 50- to 55-minute cardio session on a stair stepper, or substitute another cardio machine, swimming, or outdoor walking and running. For more information on intensity levels, flip to the introduction of this book. Do this workout today and Friday.

The following is your workout:

1. 3 minutes: Warm up at moderate pace at intensity level 5

2. 50 minutes: Step it up and be breathless and sweaty with intensity level 6 to 8

3. 2 minutes: Cool down at an intensity level of 3 to 4

# WEDNESDAY: LIFTING YOUR BOTTOM LINE WITH PILATES

This week, do two Pilates sessions with the moves from week three and add the leg exercises from these pages. Here's how it works: after The Seal exercise in week three, move right into amazing leg and butt work here with the Standing Leg Series. It should look familiar because it's the same as in previous weeks, only now you're standing to slim down and tone up from head to toe so you can show off that bikini bod! Follow the exercises in the order shown, all directions, including the breathing patterns, and shoot for 10 reps of all exercises unless I tell you differently. Start with the right leg; then, after you complete all the exercises listed in this section, switch legs.

Here's how you know you're doing the exercises correctly: your outer thigh on the standing leg will begin to heat up with a little burn and that's because the standing leg is working hard to stabilize you. In other words, you're working all the lovely muscles in your leg from your ankle to your hip. Don't forget to run through your mental and verbal checklist: head, neck, shoulders, and hips (see the introduction of this book for details). Be sure to do all the exercises with your right leg, and only then switch to your left leg and go through all the exercises again!

The following are the Pilates exercises you'll be doing today:

- Standing Sweep Kick
- Standing Beat … Beat … UP
- Standing Side Passé
- Standing Leg Circle (front and back)
- Standing Outer Thigh Lift
- Standing Booty Lift
- Standing Front Kick
- Standing Bicycle
- Standing Curtsy

By now, you should be feeling tighter and leaner—and seeing those lovely abs. Yes, the legs and butt are the last to change, but trust me, these interval exercises will deliver body results, so stick with it!

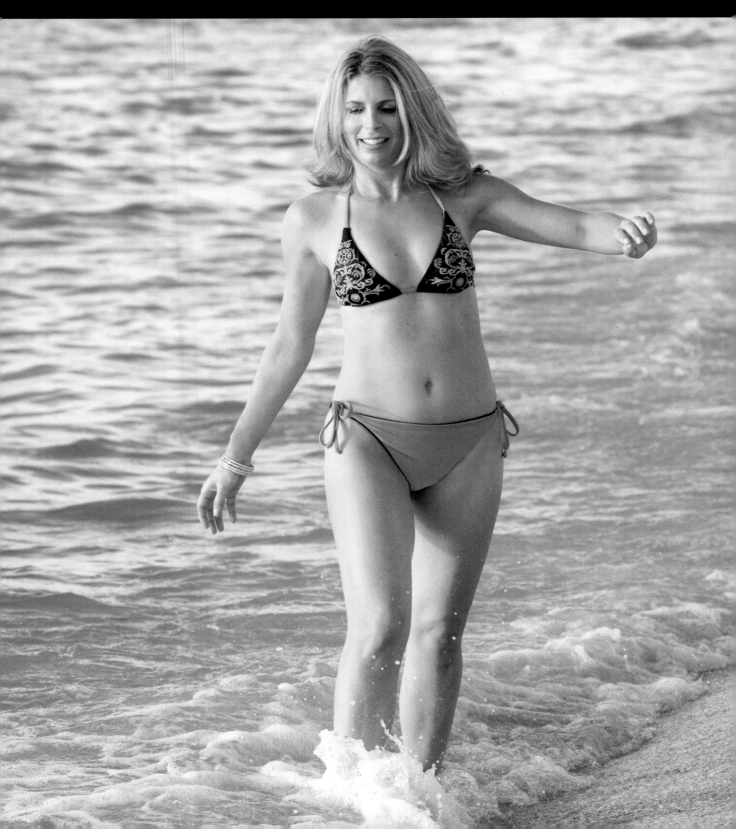

# Standing Sweep Kick

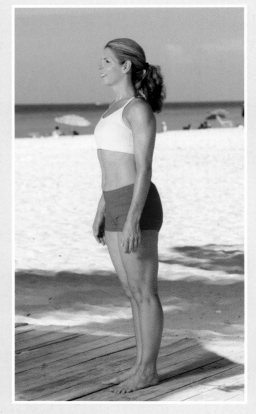

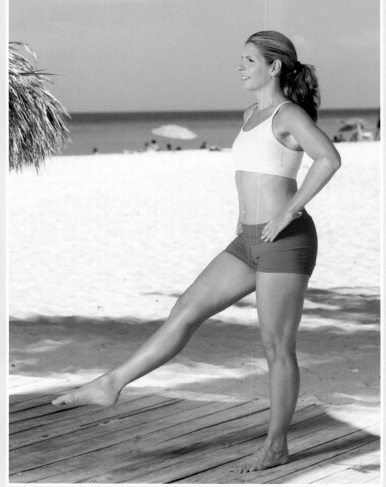

**STARTING POSITION:** Stand with your heels together and straighten your arms by your sides, in a Pilates "V." Your hip points face forward and remain even. Lift from the top of your head and drop your shoulders.

## TIPS AND TRICKS

- Don't lock or hyperextend your knees; lift from your kneecaps to turn on all the muscles in your legs-from your ankles to your hips.

- Don't arch your back as the leg swings back.

**POSITION 1:** Lift your foot off the ground, and with a straight leg inhale to kick your leg forward about hip height; add another small kick.

## THE PAYOFF:

Develops oh-so-lovely lean legs and a firm fanny.

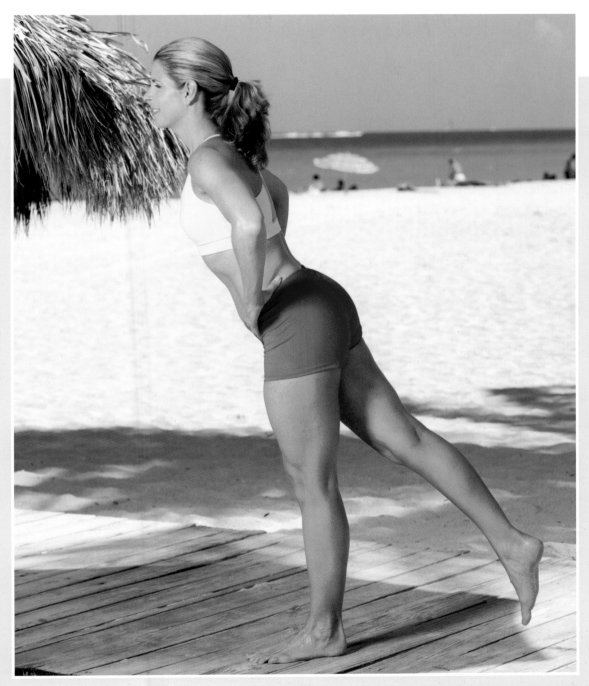

**POSITION 2:** Exhale to kick your leg back behind you; add another small kick using your booty. Your leg is moving from front to back as if you're sweeping the floor with your foot.

# Standing Beat ... Beat ... UP

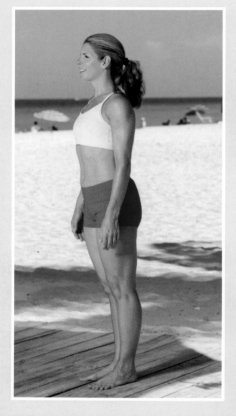

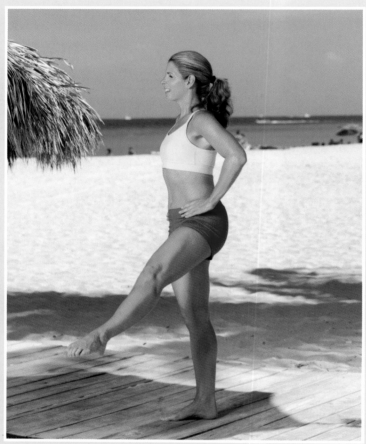

**STARTING POSITION:** Stand with your heels together and straighten your arms by your sides. Your hip points face forward and remain even. Lift from the top of your head and drop your shoulders.

**TIPS AND TRICKS**

- Don't plop your heels down; it's a small beat-beat using self-resistance so the heel of the moving leg gently touches the heel of the standing leg.

**POSITION 1:** Inhale to lift your leg to the side, letting your knee lead the way.

## THE PAYOFF:

Creates sleek and sexy inner thighs and lean legs.

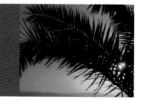

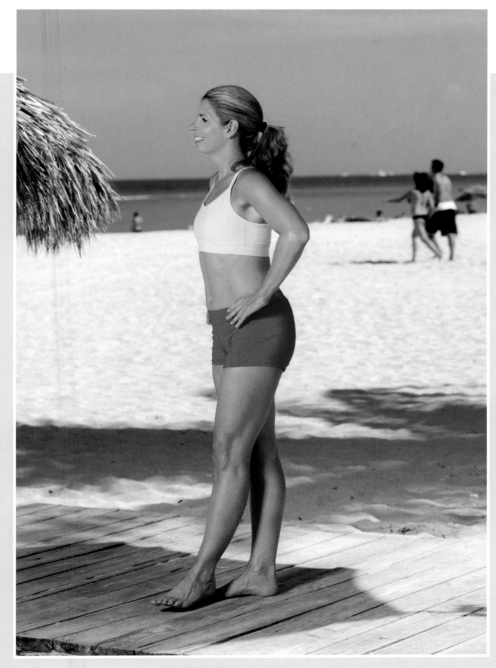

**POSITION 2:** Exhale to lower your raised heel to your standing heel, using your inner thighs. As the heel comes near the bottom heel, add a couple of quick heel beats next to the standing leg's heel.

# Standing Side Passé

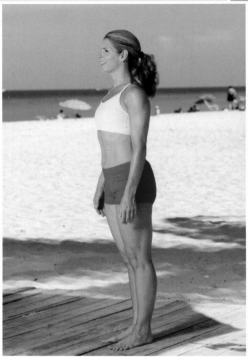

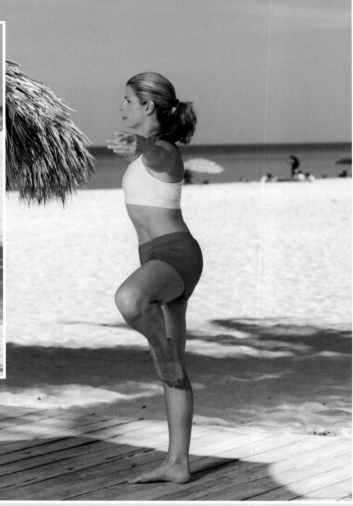

**STARTING POSITION:** Stand with your heels together and straighten your arms by your sides. Your hip points face forward and remain even. Lift from the top of your head and drop your shoulders.

## TIPS AND TRICKS

- Don't let your knee fall in; activate your butt muscles to keep your knee open to the side to open and stretch your hip.

- Don't lift your leg too high if you feel unstable; start small and then increase the range of motion.

**POSITION 1:** Inhale to open your leg to the side, so your knee turns to the side, revealing your inner thigh. Bend your knees so the heel of your foot slides along the inside of your inner thigh.

## THE PAYOFF:

Slims thighs and improves hip flexibility.

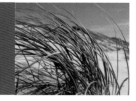

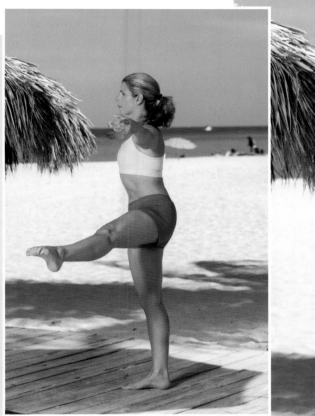

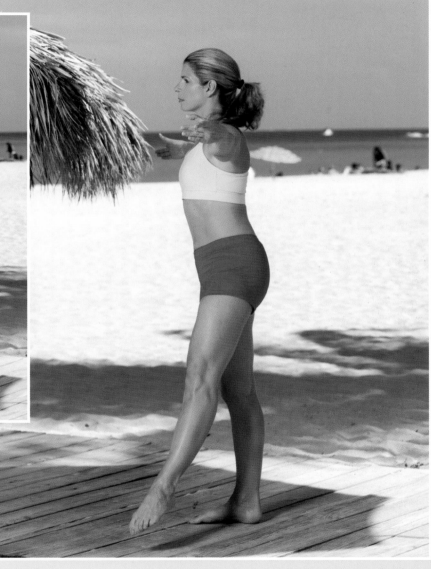

**POSITION 2:** Continue to inhale as you straighten your leg to the side.

**POSITION 3:** Exhale to lower your leg to the floor, leading with your heel to squeeze your inner thigh muscles. Repeat 5 times, and then reverse the direction of the side passé.

# Standing Leg Circle (front and back)

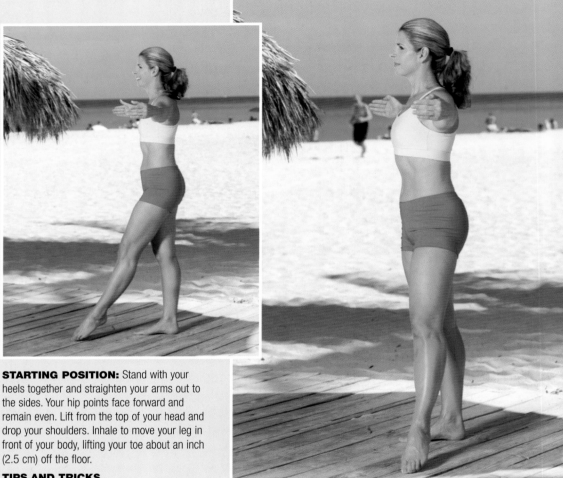

**STARTING POSITION:** Stand with your heels together and straighten your arms out to the sides. Your hip points face forward and remain even. Lift from the top of your head and drop your shoulders. Inhale to move your leg in front of your body, lifting your toe about an inch (2.5 cm) off the floor.

**TIPS AND TRICKS**

- Don't just circle from your knee, or worse, ankle; move from your butt and circle from your hips and inner thighs for yummy results.

**POSITION 1:** Exhale and make a circle on the floor with your toe. Keep your circles small so that your inner thighs touch one another with every circle. Your heel will slightly touch the heel of the standing leg. Circle your leg 10 times and then reverse direction

## THE PAYOFF:

De-dimples your thighs and butt.

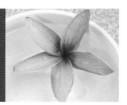

# Standing Outer Thigh Lift

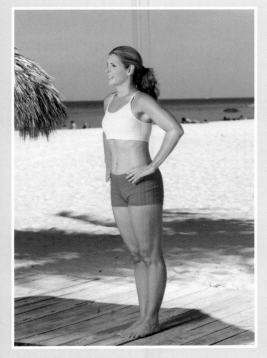

**STARTING POSITION:** Stand with your feet together in parallel and hands on your hips. Your hip points face forward and remain even. Lift from the top of your head and drop your shoulders.

**TIPS AND TRICKS**

- Don't forget to lift from your hip, keeping your toes in parallel to work your outer thighs.

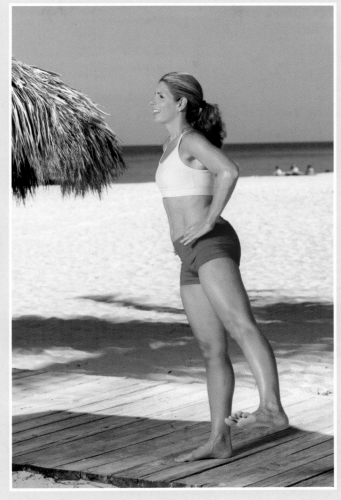

**POSITION 1:** Inhale to lift one leg to the side, with your foot absolutely parallel, and then exhale to squeeze your inner thighs and slowly lower your leg.

## THE PAYOFF:

Allows you to say bye-bye to cellulite.

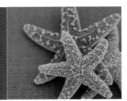

# Standing Booty Lift

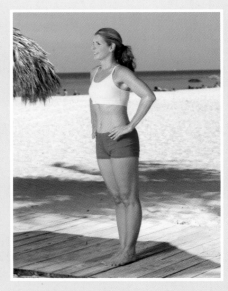

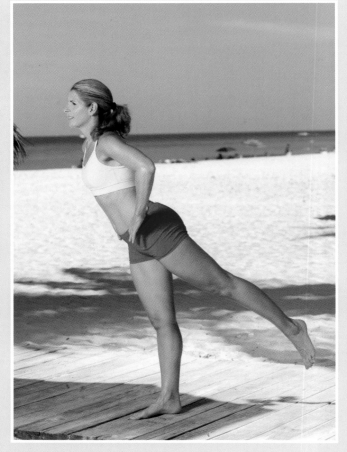

**STARTING POSITION:** Stand with your feet parallel and hands on your hips. Your hip points face forward and remain even. Lift from the top of your head and drop your shoulders.

**TIPS AND TRICKS**

- Don't sag in your belly. You may have to lean forward slightly to avoid putting needless pressure on your lower back, and to work your booty to its fullest potential.

**POSITION 1:** Inhale to lift your leg to the back, leading with your heel to engage your fanny. Exhale to lower your leg to the starting position.

## THE PAYOFF:

Lifts your bottom line.

# Standing Front Kick

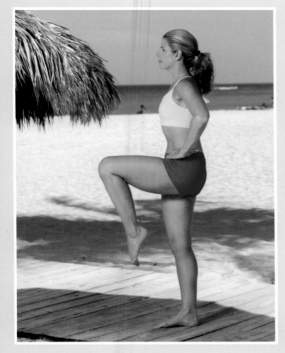

**STARTING POSITION:** Stand with your feet parallel and straighten your arms by your sides. Your hip points face forward and remain even. Lift from the top of your head and drop your shoulders. Lift your knee to hip height.

### TIPS AND TRICKS

- Don't haphazardly kick your leg out; use control to strengthen your quadriceps, or the muscles of the front thigh.

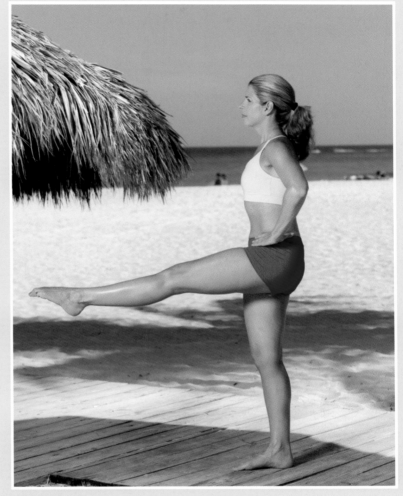

**POSITION 1:** Inhale to slowly kick your leg until it's straight, engaging your quadriceps, or the muscles of the front thigh. Exhale to bend your knee.

## THE PAYOFF:

Delivers sexy, strong legs.

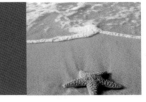

# Standing Bicycle

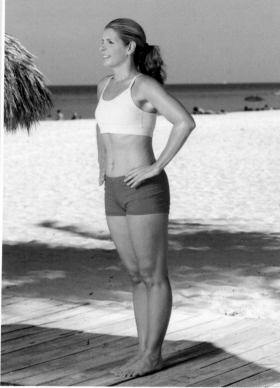

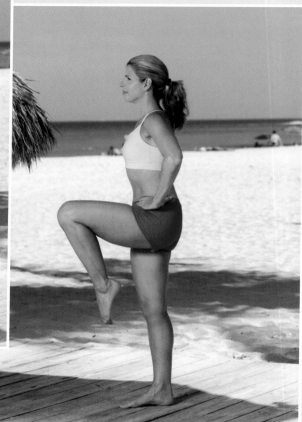

**STARTING POSITION:** Stand with your feet parallel and hands on hips. Your hip points face forward and remain even. Lift from the top of your head and drop your shoulders.

## TIPS AND TRICKS

- Don't move your pelvis as the leg moves from front to back; use your core muscles to stabilize your hips.

**POSITION 1:** Inhale to bend your knee and lift your knee to hip height.

## THE PAYOFF:

Gives you oh-so-lovely legs and a firm fanny.

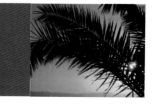

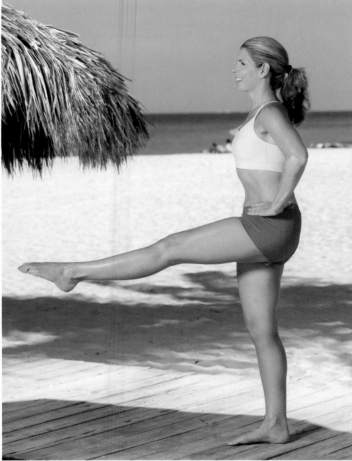

**POSITION 2:** Exhale as you straighten your leg.

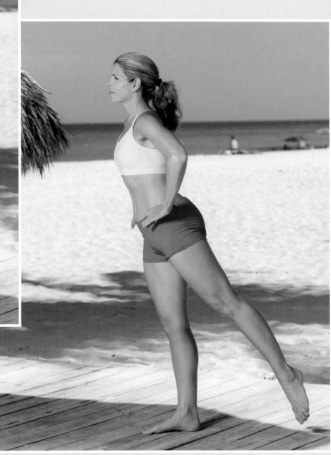

**POSITION 3:** Continue to exhale as you lower the straight leg to the floor; drag your heel across the floor and then behind you, engaging your hamstrings.

# Standing Curtsy

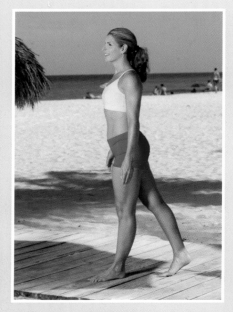

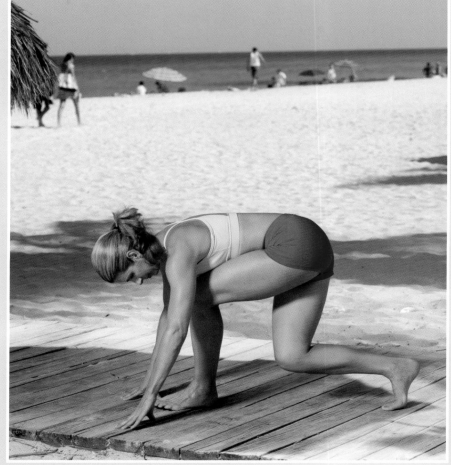

**STARTING POSITION:** From a standing position with your arms straight by your sides, bring your right leg behind your left foot, and lean slightly forward.

**TIPS AND TRICKS**

- Don't let your knee go over your toes; the majority of your body weight is in your lunge leg to challenge your hip stability and strengthen your hip.

- Don't forget to squeeze your inner thighs together for extra power.

**POSITION 1:** Inhale to bend down and place your hands on the floor while taking a big step behind so your left leg moves into a deep lunge position.

## THE PAYOFF:

Leads to major shrinkage in your thighs, plus strong legs.

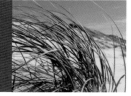

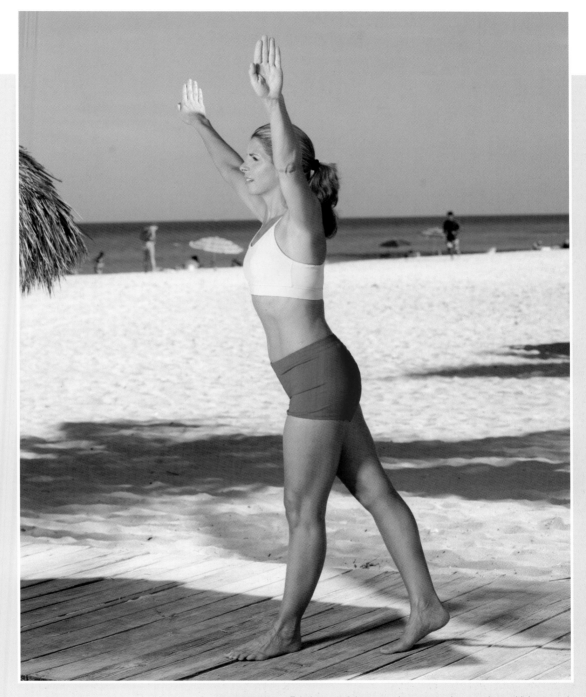

**POSITION 2:** Exhale to straighten your legs, squeezing your inner thighs together as you come to a standing position while lifting your arms over your head.

## THURSDAY: BURNING IT OFF WITH BOOT CAMP STRENGTH INTERVALS

Today, repeat Monday's boot camp workout, p. 159.

## FRIDAY: STEPPING ON IT WITH STEADY-STATE CARDIO

Today, repeat Tuesday's cardio challenge, p.170.

## SATURDAY: LIFTING YOUR BOTTOM LINE WITH PILATES

Today, repeat Wednesday's Pilates workout, p. 170.

## SUNDAY: ENJOYING YOURSELF!

You should be seeing some body (slim and trim legs and awesome abs) and booty (tighter tush) results. Try on your bikini and write down, well—what you don't see anymore!

Take today off and enjoy yourself. But let this still be a great bikini day, by adding some healthy eating habits that will get you bikini ready:

- **Nosh on apples:** Micronutrients like flavonoids keep your teeth healthy, and they naturally "brush" them, too. Apples also give you extra fiber, keeping your body healthy.

- **Eat heart-healthy fats (omega-3s):** For beautiful summer-worthy hair and skin (and you'll be showing lots of it in your bikini), eat plenty of avocados, nuts, olive oil, salmon, and flaxseed.

- **Eat more figs:** They're like the ultimate fiber food and keep your insides healthy.

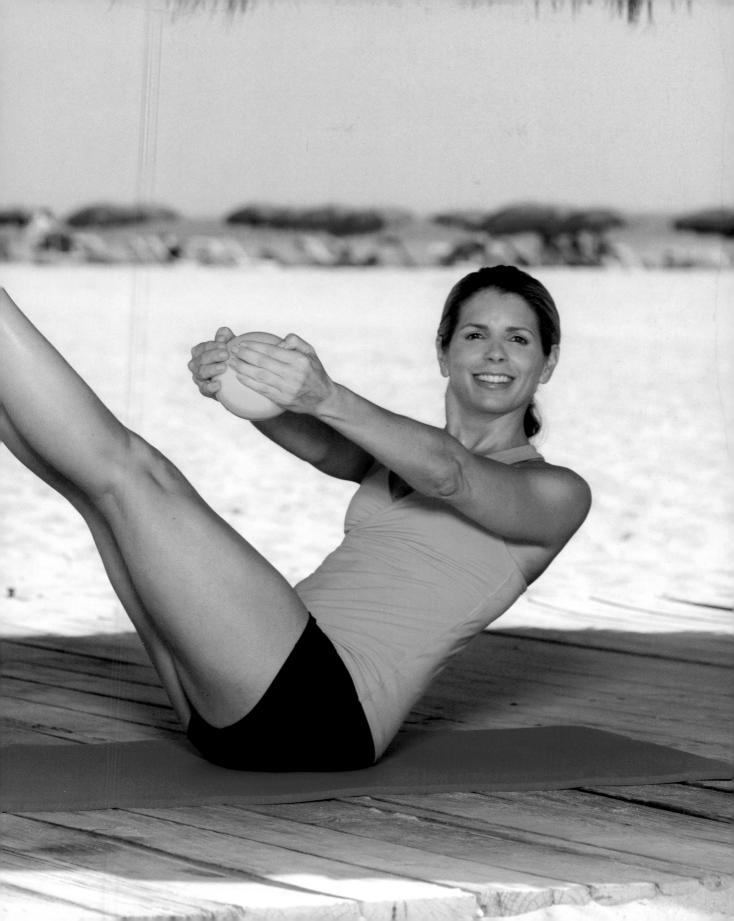

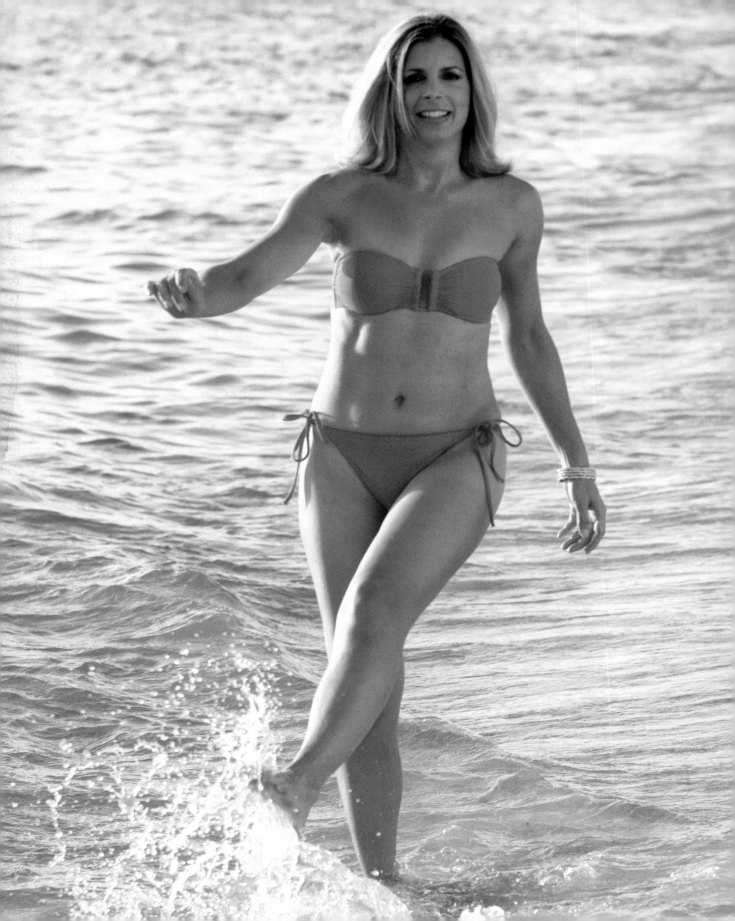

# week five

## THE BIKINI HEAT IS ON

Summer heat is right around the corner, and you can look forward to putting off your own heat, looking smoking hot in a bikini, giving everyone else heatstroke. The dramatic body changes you'll reveal by the end of the six weeks will be worth all your hard workouts. Because you're already fitter, you'll take your workouts to a new (shaky) level with balance moves that will up your "bodyliscious" quotient. Stay strong—what else would a gutsy girl wear during the hot days of summer?

| | |
|---|---|
| **MONDAY** | Fighting Fat Faster with Cardio |
| **TUESDAY** | Achieving an All Over Balance Workout |
| **WEDNESDAY** | Fighting Fat Faster with Cardio |
| **THURSDAY** | Achieving an All Over Balance Workout |
| **FRIDAY** | Fighting Fat Faster with Cardio |
| **SATURDAY** | Sculpting Beach-Worthy Abs: Pilates with Props |
| **SUNDAY** | Being Lazy! |

# week five

M T W T

| MONDAY | TUESDAY | WEDNESDAY | THURSDAY |
|---|---|---|---|
| Fighting Fat Faster with Cardio | Achieving an All Over Balance Workout | Fighting Fat Faster with Cardio | Achieving an All Over Balance Workout |

## MONDAY — Fighting Fat Faster with Cardio

1. 3 minutes: Warm up by walking 3.5 mph (5.5 kph), no grade
2. 2 minutes: Walk 3.5 to 4.0 mph (5.5 to 6.0 kph), 3 to 6 percent grade
3. 1 minute: All-out sprint 6.0 to 7.0 mph (9.5 to 11 kph), no grade
4. 1 minute: Walk 3.5 to 4.0 mph (5.5 to 6.0 kph), 3 to 6 percent grade
5. 1 minute: Run 5.0 to 5.5 mph, no grade
6. 2 minutes: Walk 3.5 to 4.0 mph (5.5 to 6.0 kph), 3 to 6 percent grade
7. 1 minute: Run 5.0 to 5.5 mph (8.0 to 8.5 kph), no grade
8. Repeat steps 2 through 7 six more times.
9. 4 minutes: Cool down by walking 3.0 to 3.2 mph (4.5 to 5.0 kph), no grade

## TUESDAY — Achieving an All Over Balance Workout

**SET 1**

Single Leg Lunge (Stationary) on Step

Ball Bridge with Chest Press

Single Leg Triceps Extension

**SET 2**

Single Leg Hip Extension with Dumbbells

Ball Bridge with Reverse Fly

Plank on Ball

**SET 3**

Single Leg Biceps Curl

Ball Bridge with Leg Curl

Push-up and Reverse Ab Curl Combination

## WEDNESDAY — Fighting Fat Faster with Cardio

1. 3 minutes: Warm up by walking 3.5 mph (5.5 kph), no grade
2. 2 minutes: Walk 3.5 to 4.0 mph (5.5 to 6.0 kph), 3 to 6 percent grade
3. 1 minute: All-out sprint 6.0 to 7.0 mph (9.5 to 11 kph), no grade
4. 1 minute: Walk 3.5 to 4.0 mph (5.5 to 6.0 kph), 3 to 6 percent grade
5. 1 minute: Run 5.0 to 5.5 mph, no grade
6. 2 minutes: Walk 3.5 to 4.0 mph (5.5 to 6.0 kph), 3 to 6 percent grade
7. 1 minute: Run 5.0 to 5.5 mph (8.0 to 8.5 kph), no grade
8. Repeat steps 2 through 7 six more times.
9. 4 minutes: Cool down by walking 3.0 to 3.2 mph (4.5 to 5.0 kph), no grade

## THURSDAY — Achieving an All Over Balance Workout

**SET 1**

Single Leg Lunge (Stationary) on Step

Ball Bridge with Chest Press

Single Leg Triceps Extension

**SET 2**

Single Leg Hip Extension with Dumbbells

Ball Bridge with Reverse Fly

Plank on Ball

**SET 3**

Single Leg Biceps Curl

Ball Bridge with Leg Curl

Push-up and Reverse Ab Curl Combination

## F S S

| FRIDAY | SATURDAY | SUNDAY |

### Fighting Fat Faster with Cardio

### Sculpting Beach-Worthy Abs: Pilates with Props

### Being Lazy!

OFF

1. 3 minutes: Warm up by walking 3.5 mph (5.5 kph), no grade

2. 2 minutes: Walk 3.5 to 4.0 mph (5.5 to 6.0 kph), 3 to 6 percent grade

3. 1 minute: All-out sprint 6.0 to 7.0 mph (9.5 to 11 kph), no grade

4. 1 minute: Walk 3.5 to 4.0 mph (5.5 to 6.0 kph), 3 to 6 percent grade

5. 1 minute: Run 5.0 to 5.5 mph, no grade

6. 2 minutes: Walk 3.5 to 4.0 mph (5.5 to 6.0 kph), 3 to 6 percent grade

7. 1 minute: Run 5.0 to 5.5 mph (8.0 to 8.5 kph), no grade

8. Repeat steps 2 through 7 six more times.

9. 4 minutes: Cool down by walking 3.0 to 3.2 mph (4.5 to 5.0 kph), no grade

**The following are the Pilates exercises you'll be doing today:**

The Hundred

Roll-up with 2-Pound Balls

Roll Over

Single Leg Circle

Rolling Like a Ball

Single Leg Stretch with 2-Pound Balls

Double Leg Stretch with 2-Pound Balls

Straight Scissor Legs with 2-Pound Balls

Double Leg Lift with 2-Pound Ball

Criss-Cross with 2-Pound Ball

Spine Stretch

Open Leg Rocker

Corkscrew

Saw with 2-Pound Balls

Swan

Single Leg Kick

Double Leg Kick

Neck Pull with Oblique Twist and 2-Pound Ball

Shoulder Bridge with One Leg

Teaser Twist with 2-Pound Ball

The Seal

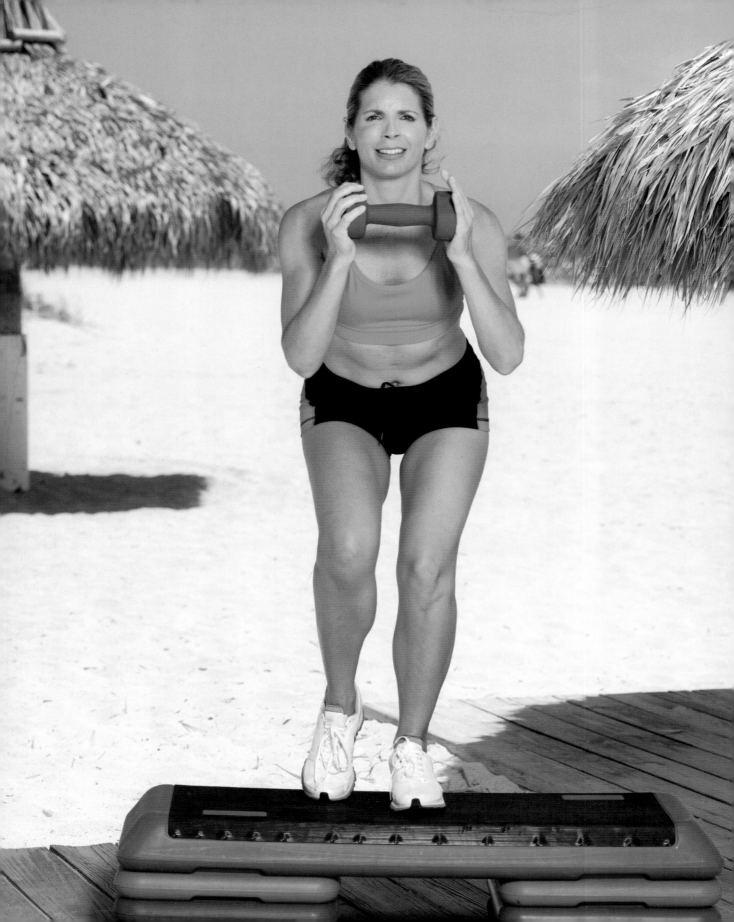

# MONDAY: FIGHTING FAT FASTER WITH CARDIO

To get bikini lean, you'll alternate between high- and low-intensity intervals to keep your heart rate up. Today, you'll do a 50- to 55-minute very high intensity workout, and it's a bit different than the previous weeks. For example, you will do an all-out sprint for 1 minute, then decrease to a walk for 1 minute, then increase to a run for 1 minute for your high-intensity intervals. (Note that "no grade" means "no incline." The grade is to add intensity. If you feel this is too difficult, just do the workout and don't worry about the grade.) If you don't have a gym membership or want to be outside, you can alternate between power walking, sprinting, and running, looking for a hill on which to do the inclines. See the introduction to this book for equivalent intensity levels if you're not using a treadmill.

The following is your treadmill workout:

1. 3 minutes: Warm up by walking 3.5 mph (5.5 kph), no grade
2. 2 minutes: Walk 3.5 to 4.0 mph (5.5 to 6.0 kph), 3 to 6 percent grade
3. 1 minute: All-out sprint 6.0 to 7.0 mph (9.5 to 11 kph), no grade (can't talk)
4. 1 minute: Walk 3.5 to 4.0 mph (5.5 to 6.0 kph), 3 to 6 percent grade (recovery)
5. 1 minute: Run 5.0 to 5.5 mph, no grade (heavy breathing)
6. 2 minutes: Walk 3.5 to 4.0 mph (5.5 to 6.0 kph), 3 to 6 percent grade (recovery)
7. 1 minute: Run 5.0 to 5.5 mph (8.0 to 8.5 kph), no grade (heavy breathing)
8. Repeat steps 2 through 7 six more times.
9. 4 minutes: Cool down by walking 3.0 to 3.2 mph (4.5 to 5.0 kph), no grade

# TUESDAY: ACHIEVING AN ALL OVER BALANCE WORKOUT

This is your last all over workout, and now you're going to test your balance and strength. Without balance and strength, you couldn't even do the simplest of tasks, such as tie your shoes. But here's the awesome part, you'll burn way more calories because you're asking a variety of muscles to work, including your core! You'll need a couple sets of dumbbells: 15 or 20 pounds (7 or 9 kg) for your legs and 8 or 10 pounds (4 or 5 kg) for your arms, plus a stability ball.

To do this all over workout you'll do 15 to 20 reps of each exercise in Set 1, and then repeat the set twice more. For example, complete 15 to 20 slow and controlled reps of the first set: Single Leg Lunge on Step, Ball Bridge with Chest Press, and Single Leg Triceps Extension. Do that set three times before moving on to Set 2, and then finish with Set 3. Total time should be about 45 minutes to 1 hour. If you're not clear on what a set or a rep is, flip to the introduction of this book. Don't forget to warm up on the treadmill for 5 minutes at 3.5 mph (5.5 kph).

**SET 1**

Single Leg Lunge (Stationary) on Step

Ball Bridge with Chest Press

Single Leg Triceps Extension

**SET 2**

Single Leg Hip Extension with Dumbbells

Ball Bridge with Reverse Fly

Plank on Ball

**SET 3**

Single Leg Biceps Curl

Ball Bridge with Leg Curl

Push-up and Reverse Ab Curl Combination

## FINDING WORKOUT BALLS

Depending on the manufacturer, stability balls come in three different sizes, but most students use a 55 cm or 65 cm. When using the ball, make sure your knees fall even with or slightly above your hips, and keep the ball at a firm intensity level. You can also find the small weighted balls at any local sporting goods store for about $7.

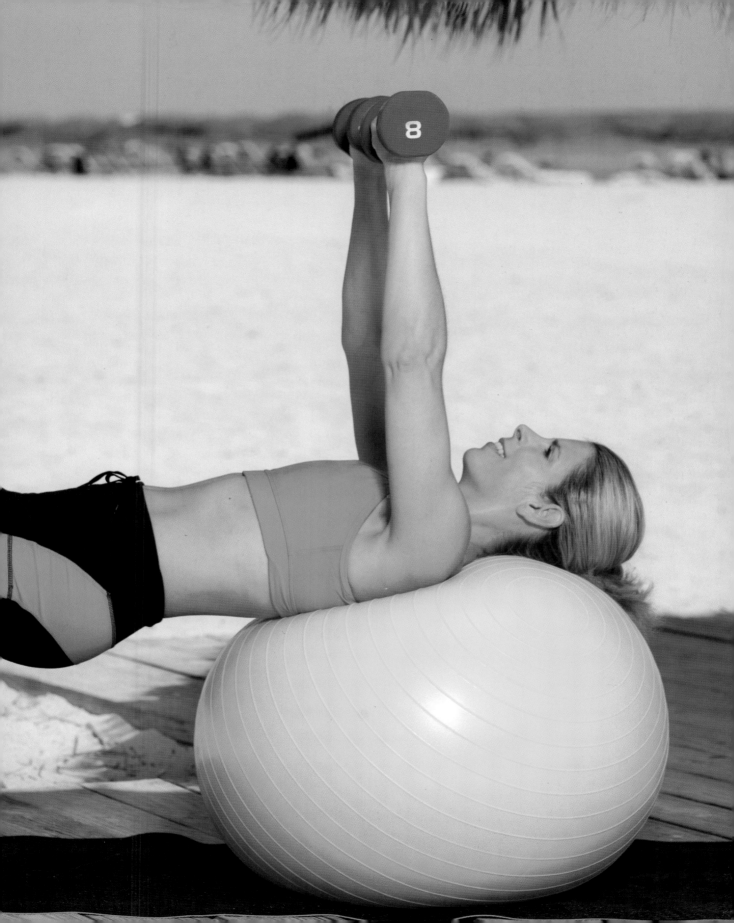

# Single Leg Lunge (Stationary) on Step

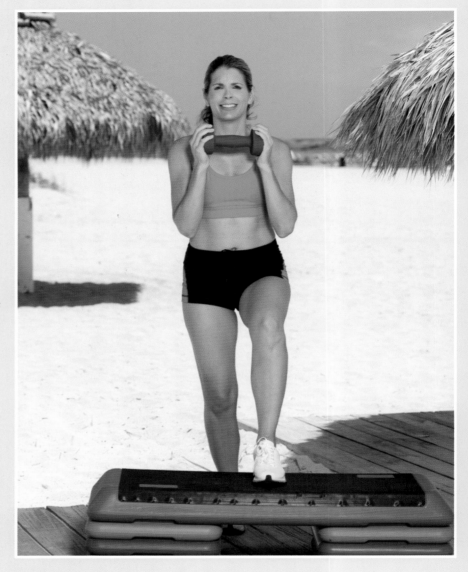

**STARTING POSITION:** Stand behind your step and place one foot on a step (about 4 rises high) or on a stairway. To ignite your core, hold an 8- to 10-pound (4 to 5 kg) dumbbell in front of your chest. Your hip points face forward and engage your abs.

**TIPS AND TRICKS**

- Don't move your leg on the step; stay in a deep lunge to challenge your stability and tone your legs and butt.

- Don't move your knee; sink deep into your hip.

- Don't round your upper back; drop the weight if you can't stay straight in your spine.

## THE PAYOFF:

Perks up your butt and slims down your legs.

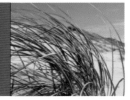

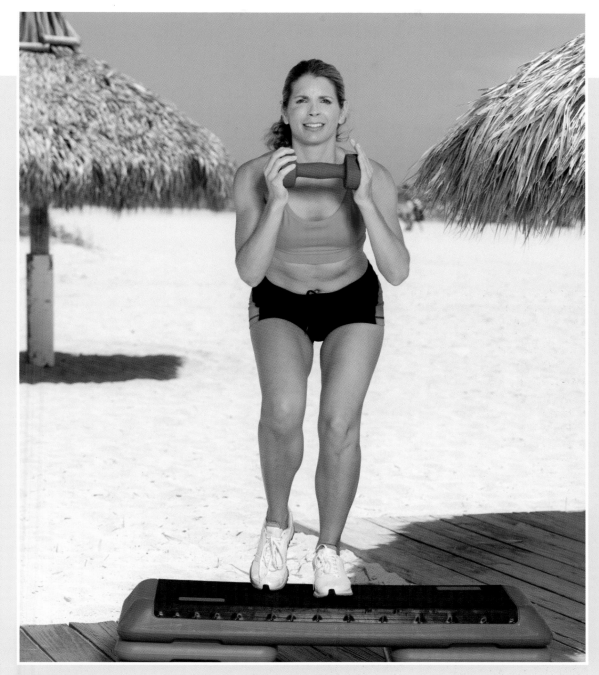

**POSITION 1:** At the same time, get into a lunge position with your foot on top of the step. Your thigh is parallel to the step as the bottom foot lifts and lowers, tapping the step. Stay in that lunge the whole time, sinking into your hip to stay stable and work your butt. Lift from the top of your head and drop your shoulders. Do 15 to 20 reps on the right leg, then do 15 to 20 reps on the left leg.

# Ball Bridge with Chest Press

REPLAY WEEK SIX

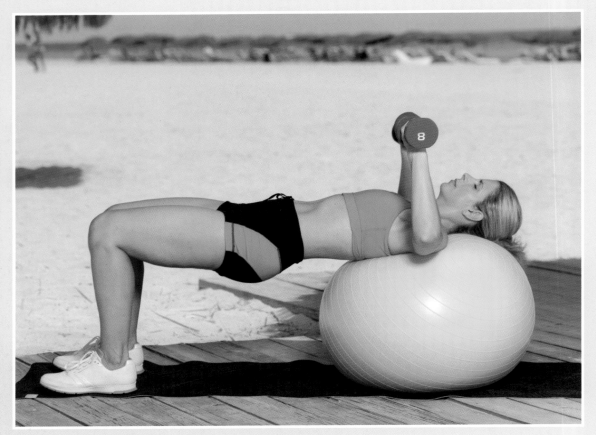

**STARTING POSITION:** Hold an 8- to 10-pound (4 to 5kg) dumbbell in each hand, sit on the center of your ball, and walk down until your upper back is on the ball. While in the bridge position, bend your elbows out to the sides of your shoulders, knuckles up.

**TIPS AND TRICKS**

- Don't sag in your booty; lift from your backside.
- Don't haphazardly lift or lower your arms; use your core and control each rep.

## THE PAYOFF:

Develops sexy curves in your chest and shoulders.

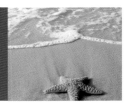

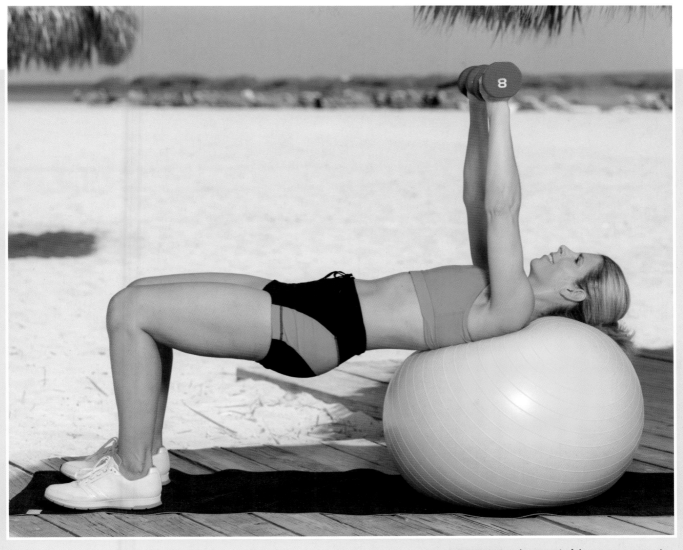

**POSITION 2:** In a count of 4, press your arms to the ceiling, then slowly lower your arms to the ball.

# Single Leg Triceps Extension

REPLAY WEEK SIX

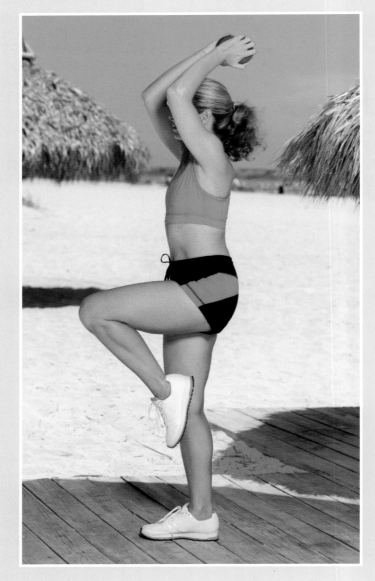

**STARTING POSITION:** Stand with feet hip width apart and hold an 8- to 10-pound (4 to 5 kg) dumbbell in both hands. Lift your arms over your head so your elbows bend forward as the weight drops behind your head, at about a 90-degree angle. Stand tall and lift your left knee to hip height.

**TIPS AND TRICKS**

- Don't bulge your abs; engage your core muscles to help you balance, especially as you lower and lift the weight to the ceiling.
- Don't look down; lengthen from the top of your head and gaze at a spot on the wall to help you balance.
- Don't swing your elbows; keep them stable to fully work your triceps.

## THE PAYOFF:

Leads to incredibly sexy arms.

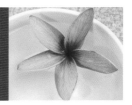

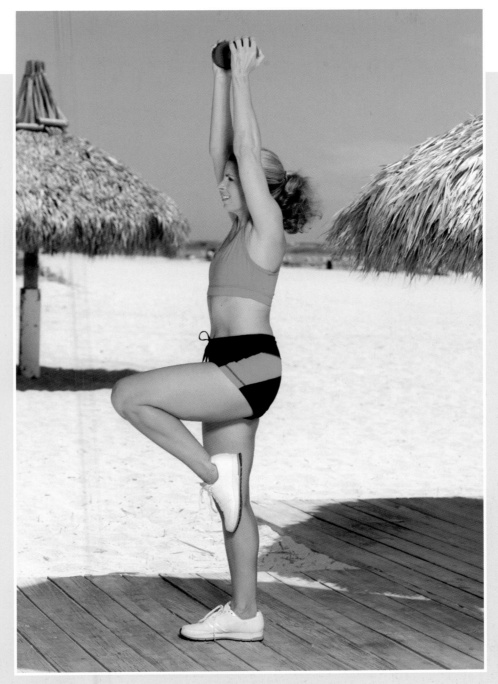

**POSITION 1:** In a count of 4, lift the dumbbell to the ceiling, then slowly lower the dumbbell. Do 10 reps on the left leg, and then 10 reps on the right.

# Single Leg Hip Extension with Dumbbells

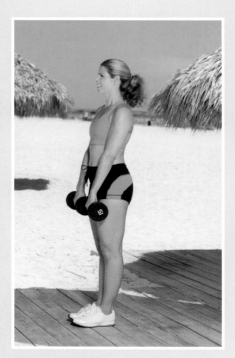

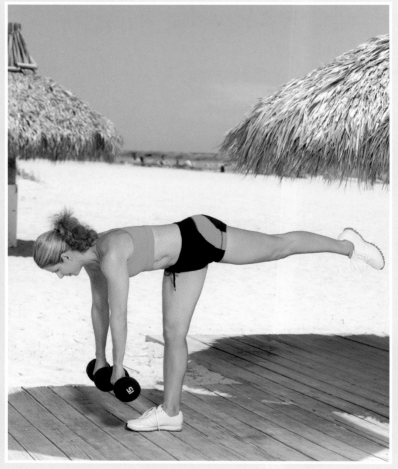

**STARTING POSITION:** Stand with feet hip width apart, with your knees straight. Hold a 15- to 20-pound (7 to 9 kg) dumbbell in each hand.

## TIPS AND TRICKS

- Don't jut your chin forward; your head follows your spine, keeping your torso completely straight.
- Don't sag your belly. Lift your navel to the sky to support your lower back. If you have a lower back injury, check with your doctor first.

**POSITION 1:** At the same time, bend at the waist, lower your chest to the floor, and lift your left leg to the ceiling, head in line with your spine. Lift your navel to the sky and then lift your torso back to a standing position. Do 12 to 15 reps on the left leg, then 12 to 15 reps on the right.

# THE PAYOFF:

Gives you a strong and stunning backside.

# Ball Bridge with Reverse Fly

REPLAY WEEK SIX

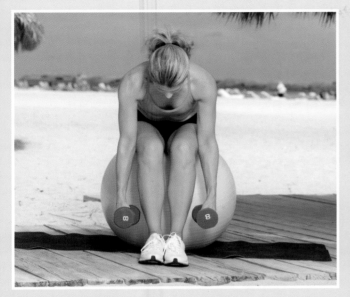

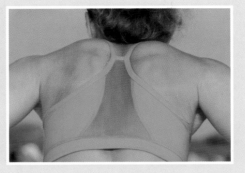

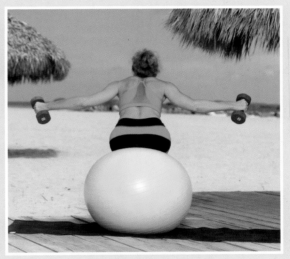

**STARTING POSITION:** Sit on the center of your ball with your knees touching, feet parallel and firmly grounded to the floor. Hold an 8- to 10-pound (4 to 5 kg) dumbbell in each hand and bend forward at the waist until your chest just about touches your thighs. Lift your breastbone slightly to help maintain a stable spine while your arms dangle by your ankles, palms down. Gaze at the floor.

### TIPS AND TRICKS

- Don't round your spine; lift from your breastbone to help keep your spine straight.
- Don't swing your arms. Instead, imagine cracking a walnut between your shoulder blades as your arms move behind you, to engage a variety of upper back muscles, including your rhomboids.
- If you can't move with control, switch to a lighter weight or don't use dumbbells at all. Your rear or posterior deltoid is usually the weakest of all your shoulder muscles, so start out with light weights.

**POSITION 1:** In a count of 4, lift your arms up and out to the sides, about shoulder height, then slowly lower your arms. Do 15 to 20 reps.

## THE PAYOFF:

Makes a sexy, sculpted back and shoulders.

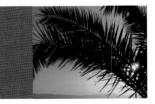

# Plank on Ball

## REPLAY WEEK SIX

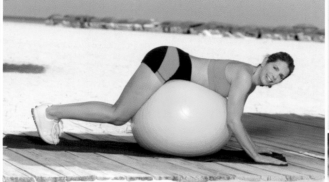

**STARTING POSITION:** Kneel in front of your ball and drape your abdomen and hips over the ball. Place your hands on the floor in front of the ball.

### TIPS AND TRICKS

- Use your legs; contract between your inner thighs for extra power—ladies, it works!

- Don't do this exercise if you have a shoulder or neck injury.

- Don't open your arms too wide; align your wrists directly under your shoulders while your shoulder blades slide down your back to create shoulder stability and work your upper back muscles. To alleviate wrist pain, consider using a pair of dumbbell weights to elevate your wrists in a neutral position.

- Don't sag your belly; if you feel pressure in your lower back, make sure your hips are not below the ball, and lift your belly button to the sky with every deep exhale.

- Don't drop your head; lengthen from the top of your head and gaze at the floor.

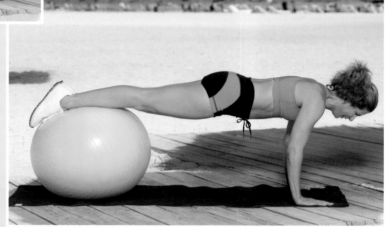

**POSITION 1:** Walk your hands out until the ball rolls toward your shins. Once you're stable, hold for 30 seconds as your body remains solid and straight, your back perfectly straight, like steel. Squeeze your thighs for inner thigh power. Focus on your exhale to engage your core and to keep you steady on the ball.

## THE PAYOFF:

Takes inches off all over and reveals a sexy core.

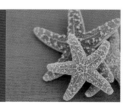

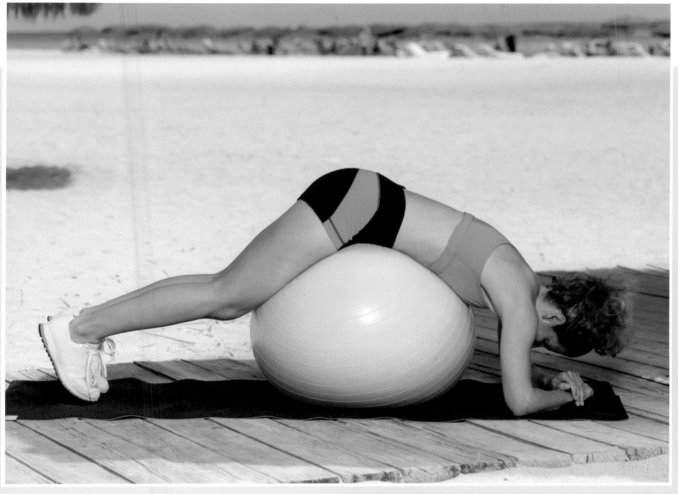

**POSITION 2:** Drape your body over the ball to stretch your lower back.

## ⭐ CORE COMPLETE

Plank is the ultimate multi muscle move: you can do a variety of levels if you're not ready for this advanced position. Putting the ball under your belly is the easiest; putting the ball under your thighs is a little harder; and putting the ball under your shins or ankles is the most difficult because gravity challenges your entire torso, creating a big core workout!

# Single Leg Biceps Curl

REPLAY WEEK SIX

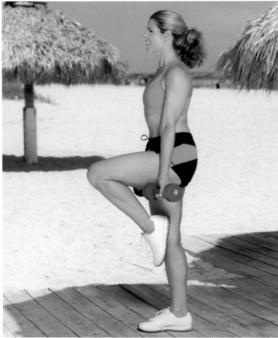

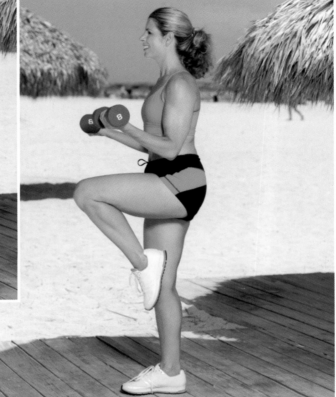

**STARTING POSITION:** Stand with feet hip width apart and hold an 8- to 10-pound (4 to 5 kg) dumbbell in each hand. At the same time, lift your left knee hip height and lower your arms by your sides. Lengthen from the top of your head to maintain a straight spine.

**TIPS AND TRICKS**

- Engage your core muscles to help you balance as you lift the weights.
- Don't look down; find a spot on the wall and gaze at it to help you balance.
- Don't swing your elbows as you curl; use smooth and controlled movements.

**POSITION 1:** In a count of 4, curl the dumbbells to your chest, then slowly lower them. Do 10 reps on the left leg, then 10 reps on the right.

## THE PAYOFF:

Sculpts sexy, strong arms.

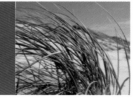

# Ball Bridge with Leg Curl

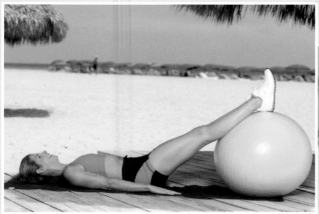

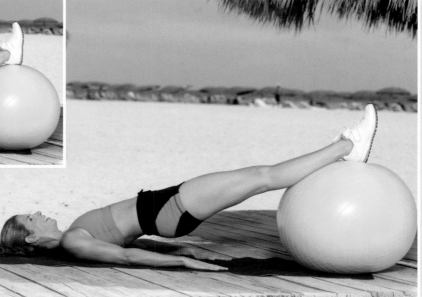

**STARTING POSITION:** Lie on your back with the ball under your knees, against the backs of your thighs so your knees are bent at a 90-degree angle. Straighten your arms by your sides, palms down.

### TIPS AND TRICKS

- Don't droop your hips; stay strong in your core and engage your butt to keep your hips even and your pelvis stable.

- Don't sag anywhere; your breastbone and pubic bone should form one line. If you feel a slight burn in the backs of your legs, or hamstrings, then don't roll the ball in as much.

- Use your arms; press the palms of your hands into the floor to help keep you steady while working your legs.

**POSITION 1:** Walk the ball out so it's under your calves. Lift your hips to the sky so your back is off the floor. Plant your heels into the center of your ball.

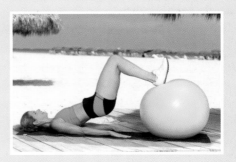

**POSITION 2:** With your heels, roll the ball toward your butt. Stay lifted in your hips as you roll it in and out. Do 15 to 20 reps.

## THE PAYOFF:

Takes inches off your backside and perks up your butt.

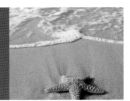

# Push-up and Reverse Ab Curl Combination

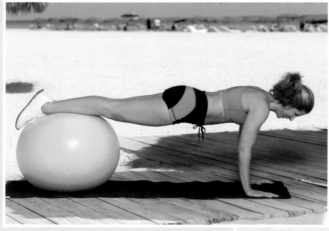

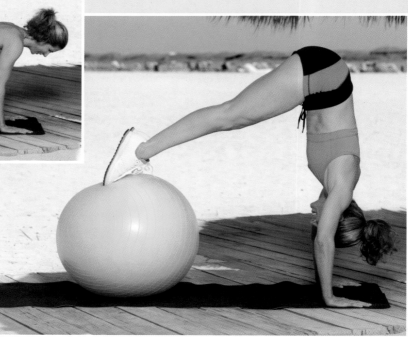

**STARTING POSITION:** Kneel in front of your ball and round your chest, abdomen, and hips over it. Place your hands on the floor in front of the ball. Walk your hands out until you are in a plank position, with your feet on the ball and your body forming a straight line. Make sure your hands are directly under your shoulders. Inhale to a plank position.

### TIPS AND TRICKS

- Breathe! Your exhale will force your abs into action and help lift your hips and support your lower back.

- Don't drop your head; look at the floor while lengthening from the top of your head so it makes a straight line with your body.

**POSITION 1:** Exhale to lift your hips to the sky so that your body forms an upside-down "V."

# THE PAYOFF:

Leads to oodles of allover tone and sexy, flat abs.

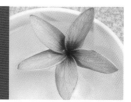

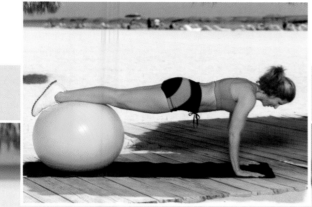

**POSITION 2:** Inhale to a plank position.

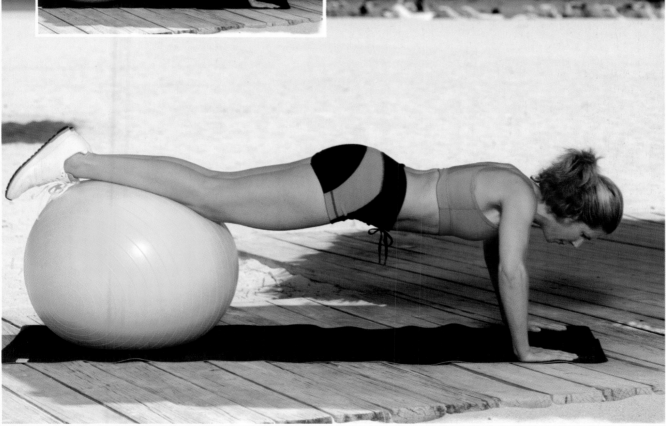

**POSITION 3:** Exhale as you bend your elbows out to the sides, lowering your body to the floor to do a push-up. Do 15 to 20 reps.

# WEDNESDAY: FIGHTING FAT FASTER WITH CARDIO

Today, repeat Monday's cardio workout, p. 193.

# THURSDAY: ACHIEVING AN ALL OVER BALANCE WORKOUT

Today, repeat Tuesday's all over balance workout, p. 194.

# FRIDAY: FIGHTING FAT FASTER WITH CARDIO

Today, repeat Monday's cardio workout, p. 193.

# SATURDAY: SCULPTING BEACH-WORTHY ABS: PILATES WITH PROPS

Come on, it's okay to be a little bit vain about your tummy! After all, your belly will be eye-catching in your bikini. Even if your stomach is of genetic good fortune and flat, you still need to keep it strong and healthy. So, this week mega watt your Pilates routine with a few fun toys: two 2-pound (1 kg) balls. The balls increase the intensity level of each exercise so you can define your sexiest, slimmest abs ever! Here's a bonus, holding the small ball works your arms, too! Follow all instructions, breathing cues, and reps.

Here's a list of the Pilates exercises you'll be doing:

- The Hundred
- Roll-up with 2-Pound Balls
- Roll Over
- Single Leg Circle
- Rolling Like a Ball
- Single Leg Stretch with 2-Pound Balls
- Double Leg Stretch with 2-Pound Balls
- Straight Scissor Legs with 2-Pound Balls
- Double Leg Lift with 2-Pound Ball
- Criss-Cross with 2-Pound Ball
- Spine Stretch
- Open Leg Rocker
- Corkscrew
- Saw with 2-Pound Balls
- Swan
- Single Leg Kick
- Double Leg Kick
- Neck Pull with Oblique Twist and 2-Pound Ball
- Shoulder Bridge with One Leg
- Teaser Twist with 2-Pound Ball
- The Seal

What's six hours a week when I'm talking about getting your most beautiful body ever? Imagine crazy sexy abs, toned legs, and a delicious derriere—no more underbutt or cellulite. You'll be fun and fearless in your bikini!

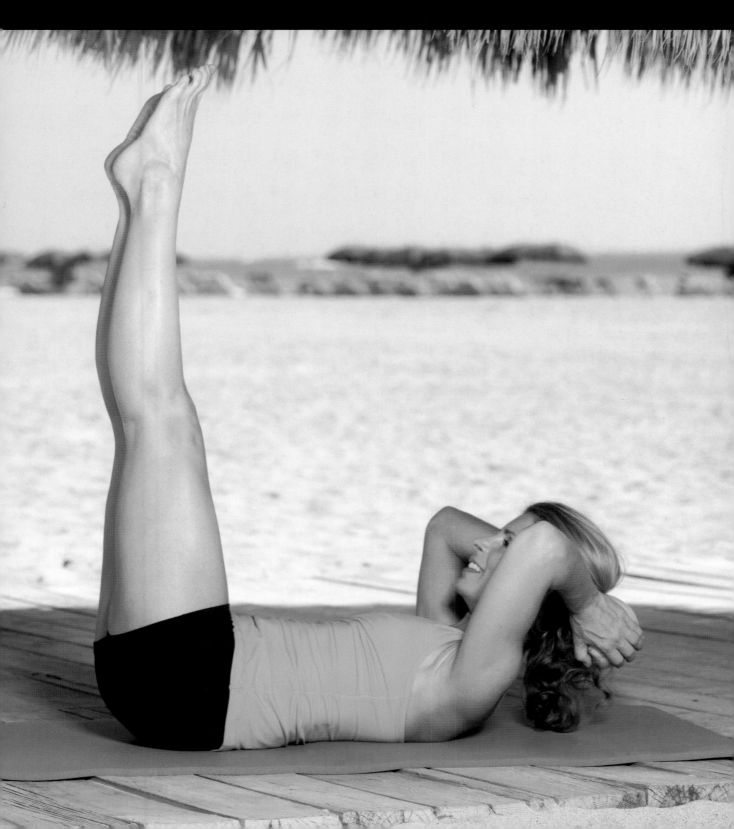

# The Hundred

REPLAY WEEKS ONE, TWO, THREE, FOUR, SIX

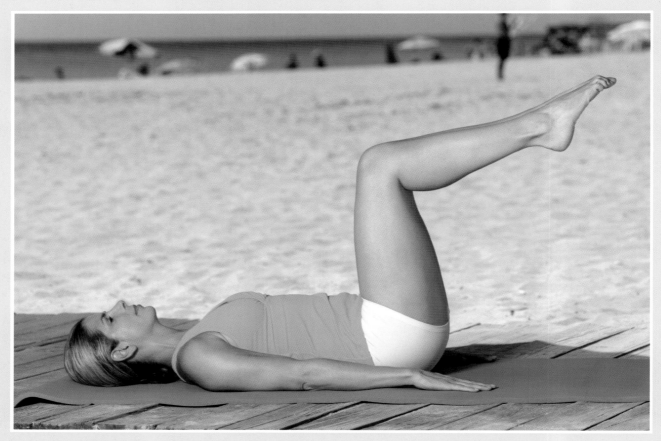

**STARTING POSITION:** Lie on your back with your knees bent, feet hip width apart. Lengthen your arms by your sides, palms down.

### TIPS AND TRICKS

- Don't bounce your torso as your arms move up and down; focus on your exhale to engage your abs, belly button to spine.

- Don't gasp for breath; keep it flowing from inhale to exhale; it's okay if you can't make it to a count of 5, do what you can.

- Don't tense your neck or clench your jaw; relax, neck tension is so not sexy! If you feel any strain, put a hand behind your head for support. Remember, strong abs can help lift your head. When they're weak, you may feel tension in your neck. Do what you can, but always protect your neck. Rest if you need it!

- Don't let your lower back come off the mat; melt your spine to the mat, using your abs to protect your lower back.

## THE PAYOFF:

Leads to sexy, strong abs and a killer figure.

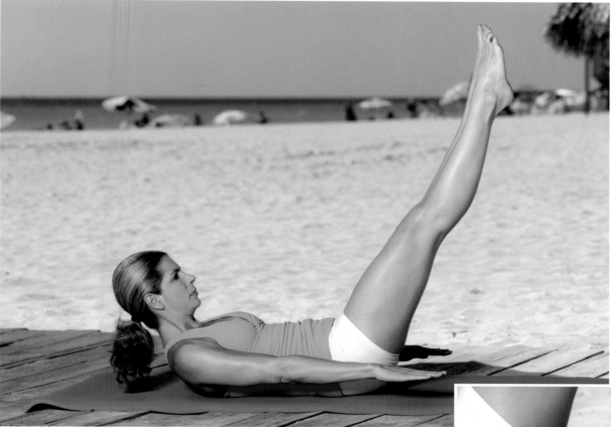

**POSITION 1:** In one motion, straighten your legs to the ceiling, feet in the Pilates "V." Curl your chin to your chest to lift your shoulders off the floor, keep your neck long. Lift and lengthen your arms past your hips, palms down, and begin pumping your arms by your sides.

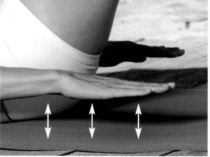

**POSITION 2:** Keeping your wrists straight, inhale to stretch your fingertips long, and pump your arms about 6 to 8 inches (15 to 20 cm) off the floor, as if you're moving your arms through thick molasses, for a count of 5, and then exhale for 5 breaths, emptying your lungs completely to drop your abs to your spine. This completes one breath cycle. Complete 10 breath cycles, thus adding up to the Hundred.

# Roll-up with 2-Pound Balls

REPLAY WEEK SIX

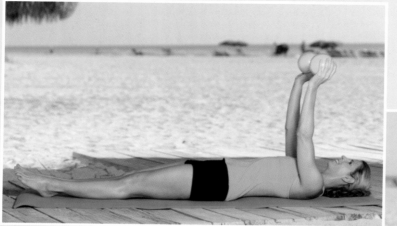

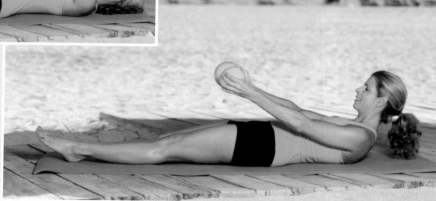

**STARTING POSITION:** Lie on your back with your legs straight, feet in a Pilates "V." Hold a ball in each hand and straighten your arms so your fingertips reach to the ceiling. Slide your shoulder blades down your back.

### TIPS AND TRICKS

- Don't lift your shoulders to your ears; instead, drop your armpits to your hips.

- Don't jerk up; if you can't roll up with control, drop the balls, bend your knees, and grab the backs of your thighs to help you.

- Don't plop down; control is crucial, so try rolling down as you press your heels away from your hips and be heavy in your heinie!

- Use your inner thighs: squeeze your legs together to streamline your inner thighs.

- Don't crane your neck; look at your belly to keep your head in line with your spine the whole time.

**POSITION 1:** Inhale to curl your chin to your chest, lifting the backs of your shoulders off the mat to look between your arms, keeping your neck long.

## THE PAYOFF:

Leads to strong, flat abs and a flexible, healthy spine.

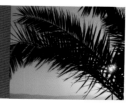

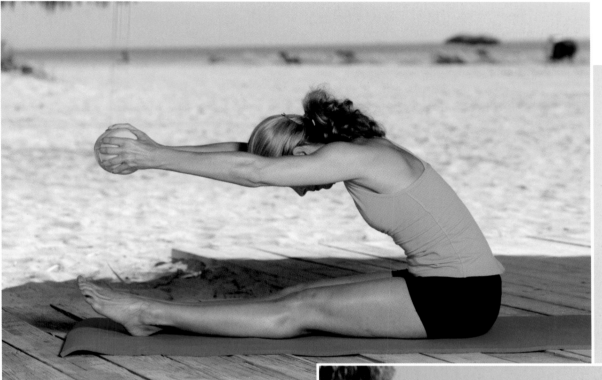

**POSITION 2:** Exhale to round over, scooping your abs. Reach your fingers past your toes and flex your feet to stretch your hamstrings.

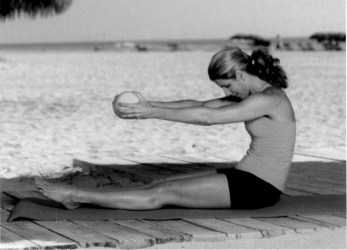

**POSITION 3:** Inhale to lift your pubic bone toward the ceiling, scooping your abs. Exhale to roll down, vertebra by vertebra, to the starting position. Imagine opening a can of sardines, curling the tin lid off. Repeat 3 to 5 times.

# Roll Over

REPLAY WEEKS THREE, FOUR, SIX

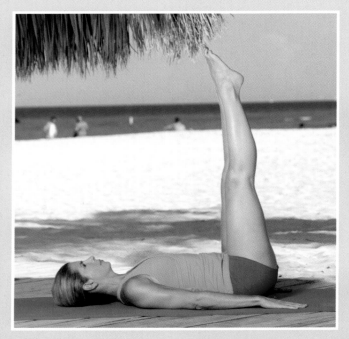

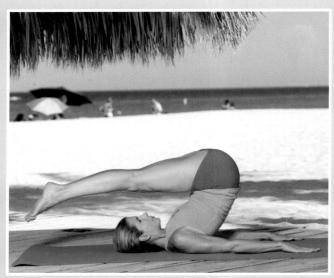

**STARTING POSITION:** Lie on your back with your legs straight at a 90-degree angle, feet in a Pilates "V." Straighten your arms by your sides, lengthening your fingertips. Slide your shoulder blades down your back.

### TIPS AND TRICKS

- Inhale to lift your legs over your head; exhale to lower your legs.

- Don't do this exercise if you have a neck or upper back injury. In addition, if you have high blood pressure or a condition called macular degeneration, check with your doctor. Exercises on your head, neck, and shoulders may not be appropriate for you.

- Don't plop down; roll down with control, pressing the backs of your arms into the mat and reaching your fingertips long to help you sink each bone into the mat.

- Don't lift your head off the mat as you roll down; scoop your abs to give you extra power.

**POSITION 1:** In one movement, press your palms into the mat and inhale to lift your hips over your head, keeping your legs closed. Hover your toes a few inches off the mat, keeping your knees directly over your eyes. Reach your fingertips long so the weight of your body doesn't land on your neck.

## THE PAYOFF:

Uncovers sexy abs and a fit, flexible spine.

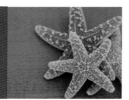

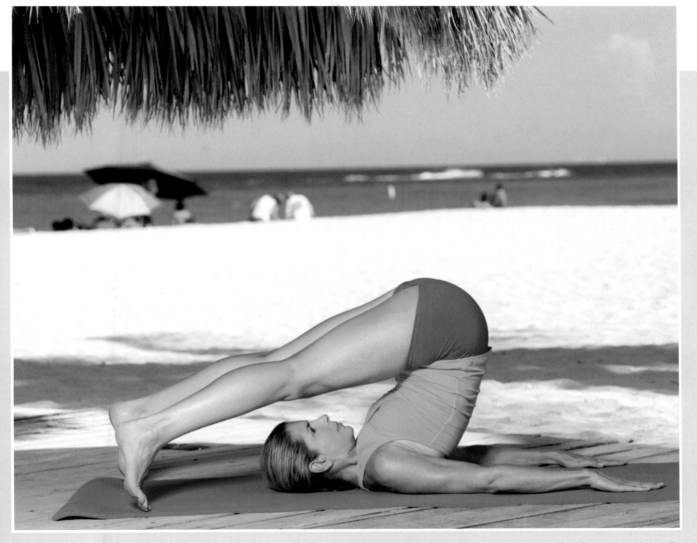

**POSITION 2:** Open your legs just past your shoulders and exhale to roll down your spine vertebra by vertebra. Feel each spinal bone pressing into the mat as you roll down until your sacrum, or the flat bone on your lower back, touches the mat. Do 3 reps with your legs closed and then 3 reps in the reverse direction, totaling 6 times. Imagine a string of pearls hitting the mat one at a time.

# Single Leg Circle

REPLAY WEEKS TWO, THREE, FOUR, SIX

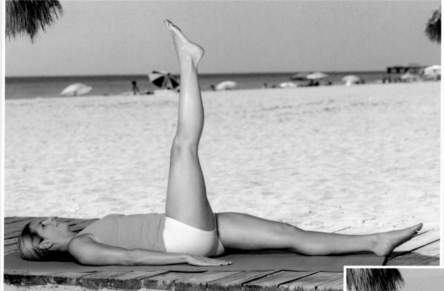

**STARTING POSITION:** Lie on your back with your left leg straight on the floor while your right leg is at a 90-degree angle, toes reaching long to the ceiling. Straighten your arms by your sides, palms down. Drop the backs of your shoulders against the mat, and slide your shoulder blades down your back.

**TIPS AND TRICKS**

- Don't rock your hips from side to side as the leg circles; fire up your core and keep your circles small at first.
- Press the palms of your hands, the backs of your arms, and the back of your head firmly into the mat, which will help stabilize you.
- Don't forget to exhale deeply to stabilize your torso and strengthen your abs.

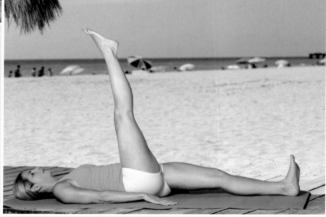

**POSITION 1:** Press your left heel into the mat and inhale to lift your right leg with your toes pointing to your nose.

## THE PAYOFF:

Develops sexy, flat abs and takes inches off your thighs.

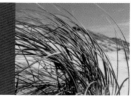

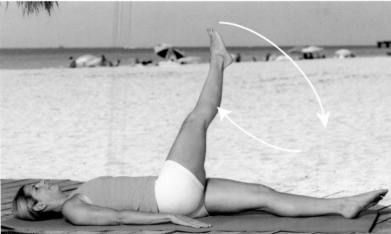

**POSITION 2:** Exhale to move the right leg across your body, inner thighs active.

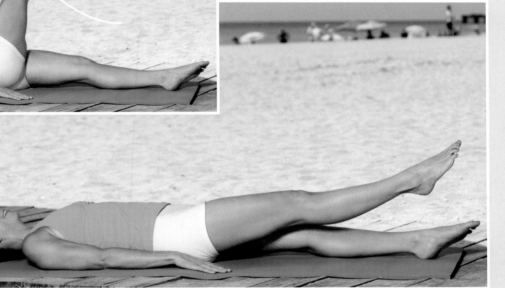

**POSITION 3:** Continue to exhale while moving your right leg to the opposite foot.

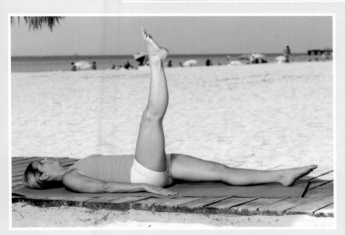

**POSITION 4:** Continue to exhale and circle your leg so it ends up at your nose. Inhale and pause slightly before circling your leg again. Imagine a string pulling your big toe to the ceiling to lengthen your leg as you circle it. Repeat 5 leg circles, and then reverse the circle for 5. Repeat with the left leg.

# Rolling Like a Ball

REPLAY WEEKS ONE, TWO, THREE, FOUR, SIX

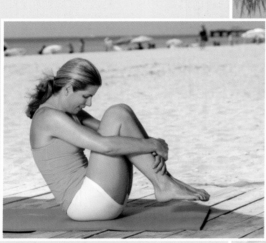

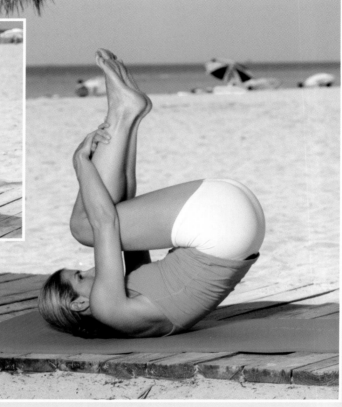

**STARTING POSITION:** Sit at the edge of the mat and slide your booty to your heels. Wrap your arms around your legs, elbows out to the sides. Place your hands on your shins, and cross them at the wrists. Your heels stay close to your bottom. Lower your head between your knees so your spine is rounded, belly button to your spine. Lift your toes about 2 inches (5 cm) off the floor. Use your abs to balance before rolling back.

**TIPS AND TRICKS**

- Don't roll on your neck; it's about lifting your fanny to the ceiling and keeping active in your belly so you roll only on your upper back.
- Don't lift your shoulders; instead, drop your armpits to your hips.

**POSITION 1:** Inhale to roll back to the middle portion of your back. Stay rounded and scoop your abs so you don't roll back onto your head. Exhale to roll up, lifting through your pelvic floor and scooping your abs for extra power. Repeat 8 to 10 times.

## THE PAYOFF:

Leads to a healthy, strong, flexible spine.

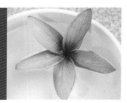

# Single Leg Stretch with 2-Pound Balls
REPLAY WEEK SIX

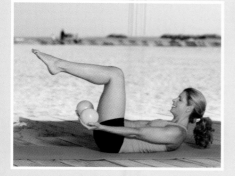

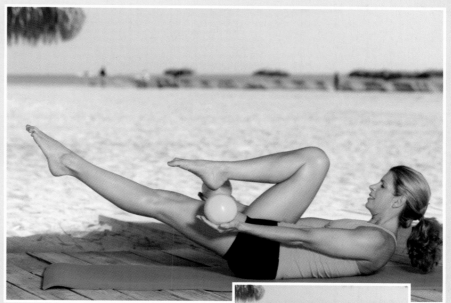

**STARTING POSITION:** Lie on your back with your knees to your chest. Hold a ball in each hand as you curl your chin to your chest to lift your shoulders off the mat. Straighten your arms by your sides.

### TIPS AND TRICKS

- Don't rock from side to side as you move your legs; engage your abs to stay stable in your torso.
- Don't bend your knees; as you move your legs away from your torso, stretch them as far a possible.
- Don't look at the ceiling; look between your thighs to maintain proper head placement and to work those abs.

**POSITION 1:** In one motion, inhale to bring your right knee to your chest, pulsing twice, while straightening your left leg so your toes are in line with your nose, or lower your leg if you want a more intense belly challenge.

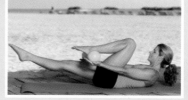

**POSITION 2:** Continue to inhale and switch legs, bringing your left knee to your chest while straightening your right leg, pulsing twice. This is one rep. Exhale to switch legs to bring your right knee to your chest while straightening your left leg; continue exhaling to switch legs to bring your left knee to your chest while straightening your right leg. Repeat 5 to 10 times.

## ⭐ THE FIVES WITH 2-POUND BALLS

Remember that The Fives (Single Leg Stretch, Double Leg Stretch, Straight Leg Scissors, Double Leg Lift, and Criss-Cross) are done in order, one right after another, to challenge all your abdominal muscles. Don't rest in between exercises, challenge your belly to do more and more and do 5 to 10 repetitions of each. The balls you're using today ramp up work for your belly, so if you feel any neck strain, drop the balls!

## THE PAYOFF:

Develops flat, sexy, strong abs.

# Double Leg Stretch with 2-Pound Balls

REPLAY WEEK SIX

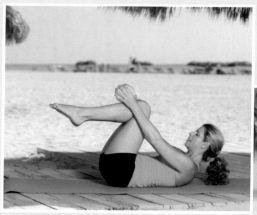

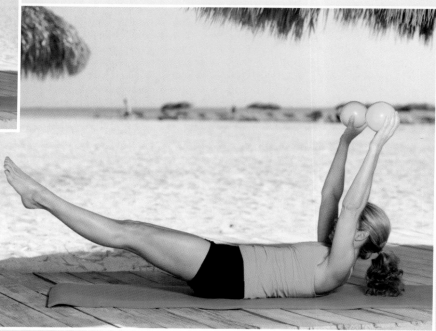

**STARTING POSITION:** Lie on your back with your knees to your chest and hold a ball in each hand, near your shins. Curl your chin to your chest and lift your head, neck, and upper back off the mat.

### TIPS AND TRICKS

- Don't look at the ceiling; keep your chin to your chest and look between your thighs at all times. If you still feel tension, your abs might not be strong enough yet. Drop the balls, rest your head on the mat, and move it from side to side between the two exercises.

- Don't bounce, jerk, or lift your lower back from the mat while your arms and legs move; your arms and legs are challenging your abs, so use them, belly button to spine the whole time.

- Don't arch your back as your legs move away from your torso; keep your back flat against the mat the whole time. If you can't maintain your back flat on the mat, lengthen your legs to the ceiling to reduce the stress on your lower back.

**POSITION 1:** In one motion, inhale to straighten your legs and reach your arms over your head; begin to circle them behind you and around. Exhale to finish the circle, then use your abs to bring your knees to your chest and tap the balls to your shins. Repeat 5 to 10 smooth, flowing stretches.

## THE PAYOFF:

Leads to crazy-strong, flat abs.

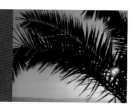

# Straight Scissor Legs with 2-Pound Balls

REPLAY WEEK SIX

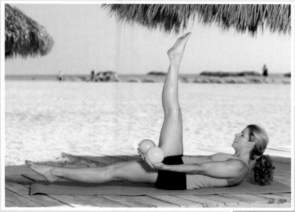

**STARTING POSITION:** Lie on your back with straight legs at a 90-degree angle and hold a ball in each hand. Straighten your arms by your sides, lift your shoulders off the mat, and curl your chin to your chest. Drop your left leg to the floor so your toes are in line with your nose while keeping your right leg at a 90-degree angle. Inhale to pulse your right leg to your forehead.

### TIPS AND TRICKS

- Don't strain your neck; your neck muscles may give out if you don't have the belly strength. Drop the balls, clasp your hands, and place them behind your head for support while you keep your legs moving. If you still feel any strain, take a break.

- Don't bounce your torso; establish a continuous smooth tempo, focusing on your breath. Also, if you don't have the hamstring flexibility, it may be difficult to straighten your legs, so bend your knees. Eventually, you'll get there!

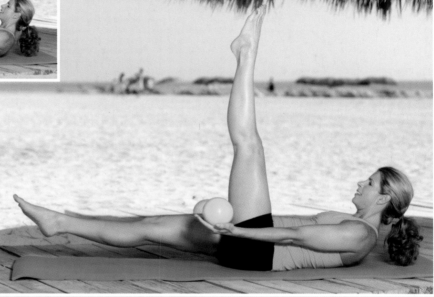

**POSITION 1:** Switch legs in a scissor like motion and exhale to pulse your left leg to your forehead. Imagine scissoring your legs as if a piece of glass were between your legs, so you're holding your legs slightly apart. Repeat 5 to 10 times.

## THE PAYOFF:

Uncovers lovely, flat abs.

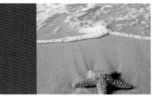

# Double Leg Lift with 2-Pound Ball

REPLAY WEEK SIX

**STARTING POSITION:** Lie on your back with straight legs lengthening to the ceiling at a 90-degree angle. Hold a ball, clasp your hands behind your head for support, and open your shoulders so you can see your elbows at your sides.

**TIPS AND TRICKS**

- Don't lift your lower back off the mat; only lower your legs without feeling this in your lower back. If you can't keep your back on the mat, bend your knees and dip your toes in the water. Don't strain your lower back.

- Don't forget to scoop, scoop, and scoop your abs.

## THE PAYOFF:

Leads to stunning abs.

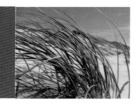

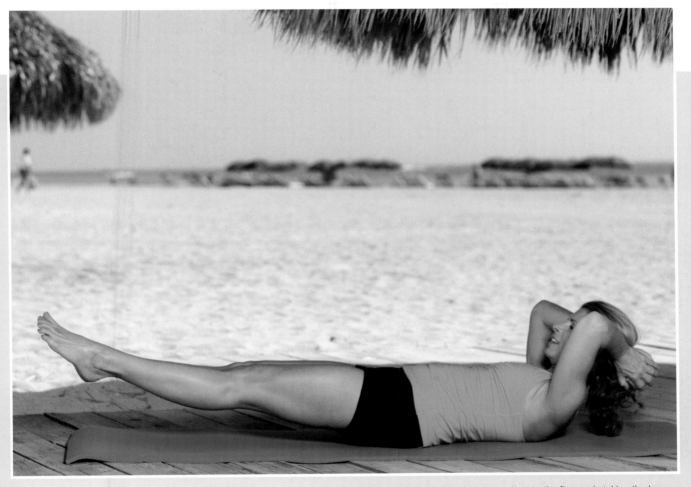

**POSITION 1:** Inhale to lower your legs to the floor, only taking the legs as low as your back is anchored to the mat: no strain, no arch, no bulge! Exhale to lift your legs to a 90-degree angle, exhaling out every last breath to drop your belly button to your spine. Imagine that a low seat belt is tightly fastened around your lower belly, from hip bone to hip bone, to feel your lower belly muscles, or transverse. Repeat 5 to 10 times.

# Criss-Cross with 2-Pound Ball

REPLAY WEEK SIX

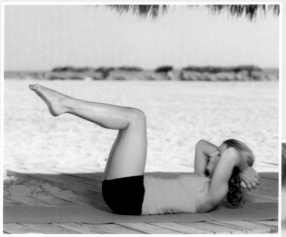

**STARTING POSITION:** Lie on your back with your knees bent at a 90-degree angle. Hold a ball, clasp your hands behind your head, and lift your shoulders off the mat.

**TIPS AND TRICKS**

- Inhale as you twist from the waist; exhale as you twist the opposite way. Imagine your ribs tightening around your belly.

- Wring out your lungs with every exhale to get that yummy oblique work. Deepen your twist on every set; your elbow reaches past the knee while you look behind you. Slow down the tempo and hold the twist—it's killer!

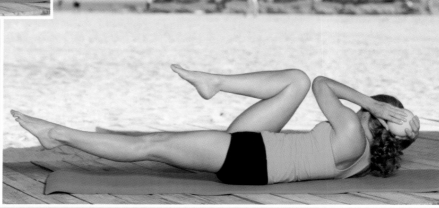

**POSITION 1:** Straighten your left leg so it's about nose level, toes in line with your nose while your right knee nears your chest. Inhale to twist from your bottom rib so your torso moves your left elbow to your right knee, armpit to knee.

## THE PAYOFF:

Scorches your love handles.

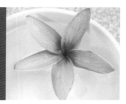

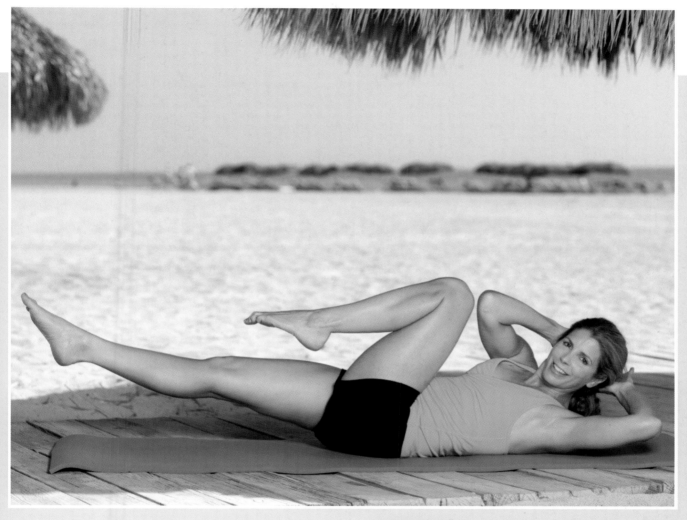

**POSITION 2:** Exhale to twist the other way, right elbow to left knee. Repeat 5 to 10 times.

# Spine Stretch

REPLAY WEEKS ONE, TWO, THREE, FOUR, SIX

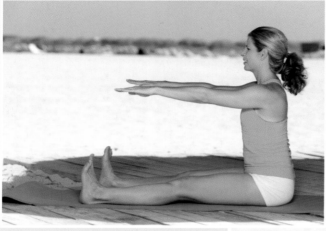

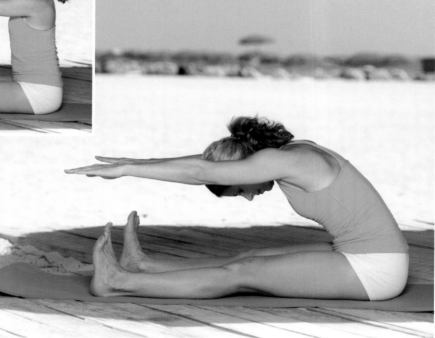

**STARTING POSITION:** Sit on your mat with your legs straight, a little wider than shoulder width apart, feet flexed. Lift your arms so they're parallel to your legs. Lift your belly button to your spine. Inhale to grow tall in your spine.

**TIPS AND TRICKS**

- Don't move your lower body; turn on your hamstrings and flex your feet as you round over.
- Don't stretch forward; scoop your abs to stretch your spine and round over. You may feel a lovely hamstrings stretch, too.
- Don't slump in your lower back; sit on top of your butt bones, as though you were sitting on hot rocks.

**POSITION 1:** Exhale to lower your chin to your chest and round over. As your fingertips stretch past your toes, scoop your abs to feel the stretch in your lower back. Imagine a mean, ugly porcupine with long, sharp needles under your belly—scoop, scoop, scoop. Inhale to roll up, vertebra on top of vertebra. Repeat 3 to 5 stretches.

## THE PAYOFF:

Leads to a healthy, flexible spine.

# Open Leg Rocker

REPLAY WEEKS THREE, FOUR, SIX

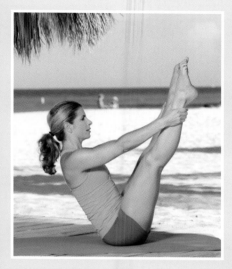

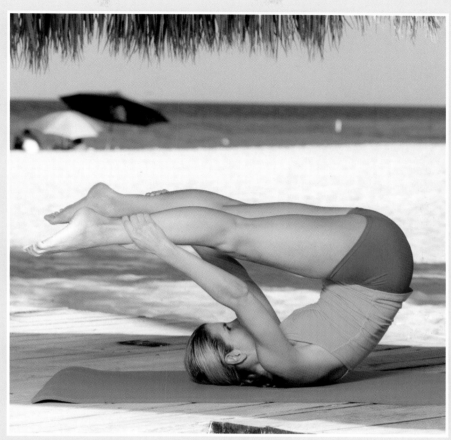

**STARTING POSITION:** Sit at the edge of the mat and slide your heels to your booty. Move your pubic bone to the ceiling and scoop your abs. Hold this scoop and then straighten your legs to make a "V." Your legs are a little wider than shoulder width apart. All limbs are straight, and your chin is on your chest.

## TIPS AND TRICKS

- Keep active in your belly and you'll be able to balance better.

- Don't roll onto your neck; roll back to your upper back by scooping your abs. If you come up too quickly or flop to one side, slightly bend your knees and scoop. It's all about focus, balance, and control.

- Use your breath as you roll up; squeeze every ounce of air out to protect your lower back. Engage your pelvic floor to give you more power.

**POSITION 1:** Inhale to roll back, making sure your weight lands on your shoulders; the top of your head never touches the mat. Exhale to roll up, scoop, scoop, and scoop to a balanced "V" position. Imagine a rocking chair; feel the rhythm of it rocking back and forth. Repeat 5 to 8 times.

## THE PAYOFF:

A 100-percent belly strengthener that leads to flat, sexy abs.

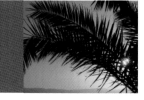

# Corkscrew

REPLAY WEEKS ONE, TWO, THREE, FOUR, SIX

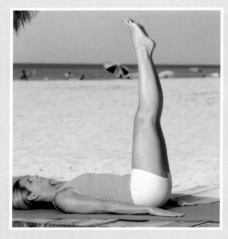

**STARTING POSITION:** Lie on your back with your legs straight at a 90-degree angle, feet in a Pilates "V." Straighten your arms by your sides, pressing the palms of your hands into the mat. Slide your shoulder blades down your back.

**TIPS AND TRICKS**

- Don't lift your head or shoulders off the mat; keep your circles small so you can maintain good form until you get strong enough.

- Don't separate your legs; squeeze your inner thighs to give you lots of power!

- Don't forget to use the power of your arms by pressing into the mat to lift your hips.

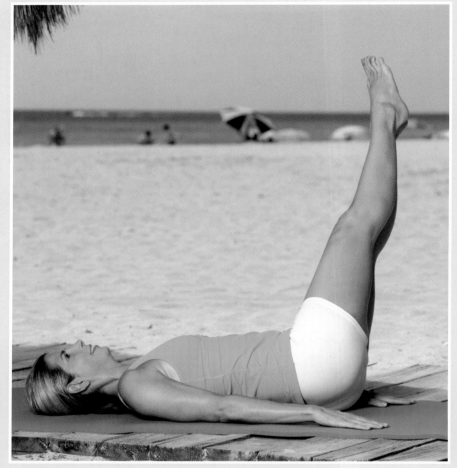

**POSITION 1:** Make a small circle with your legs to the left, letting the right hip come off the mat slightly. Keep your knees and ankles together the entire time.

## THE PAYOFF:

Scorches those love handles.

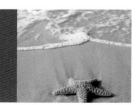

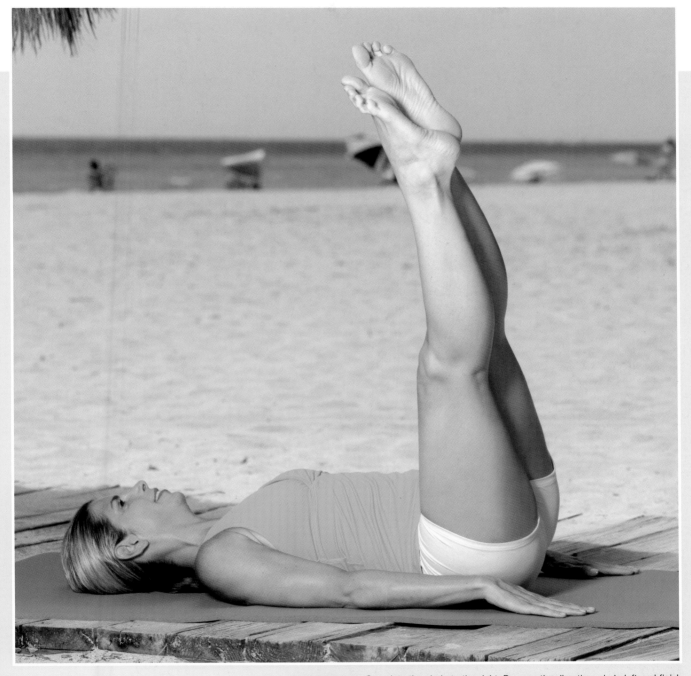

**POSITION 2:** Complete the circle to the right. Reverse the direction, circle left and finish right; that's one complete set. Imagine a string pulling your toes to the ceiling, so lengthen your legs away from your hips, keeping your knees and ankles together. Do 3 to 5 circles.

# Saw with 2-Pound Balls

REPLAY WEEK SIX

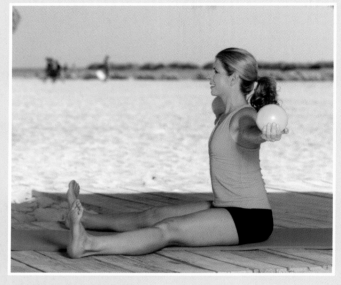

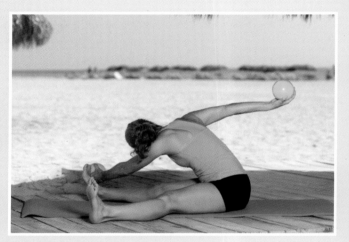

**STARTING POSITION:** Sit tall on the mat with your legs straight and a little wider than shoulder width apart, feet flexed, and hold a ball in each hand. Lift your arms out to the sides of your body, and reach your fingertips long, palms up. Inhale to grow tall in your spine, lifting your ribs slightly up off your pelvis to initiate the twist.

## TIPS AND TRICKS

- Don't bounce as you twist; it's a lengthening from your waist as you reach your arms father apart.

- Don't do any rotation if you have a back injury; please ask your doctor if "rotation" or "twisting" is appropriate for you.

- Don't slump in your lower back; sit on top of your butt bones, as if you were sitting on hot rocks!

- Don't shift or move your hips in the twist. This twist comes from the last rib on your rib cage (your ribs tighten around your stomach, using your abs). Lift up from your hips, then turn your chest and your belly button will follow.

- Don't turn your knees or feet in; keep your legs active and your knees facing up to the ceiling.

**POSITION 1:** Exhale to reach your left hand to your right foot and past the pinky toe. Imagine your left pinky finger "sawing" off your right pinky toe while your left ear moves closer to your right knee. Pulse for 3 counts while stretching your right hand behind you, palm up. With each pulse, twist a little farther, exhaling every ounce of air out of your lungs. Inhale to return to the starting position, sitting taller in your spine, and twist the other way.

# THE PAYOFF:

Gives you a stunning waist and strong obliques.

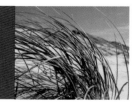

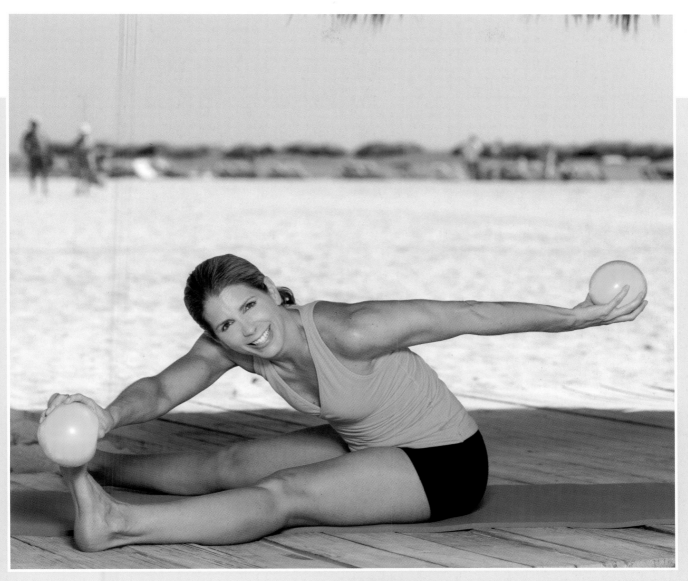

**POSITION 2:** Exhale to reach your right hand to your left foot and past the pinky toe. Imagine "sawing" off your pinky toe while your right ear moves closer to your left knee. Pulse for 3 counts while stretching your left hand behind you, palm up. With each pulse, twist a little farther, exhaling every ounce of air out of your lungs. Inhale to return to the starting position, sitting taller in your spine. Repeat 3 to 5 times.

# Swan

REPLAY WEEKS ONE, TWO, THREE, FOUR, SIX

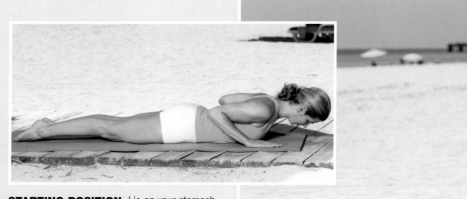

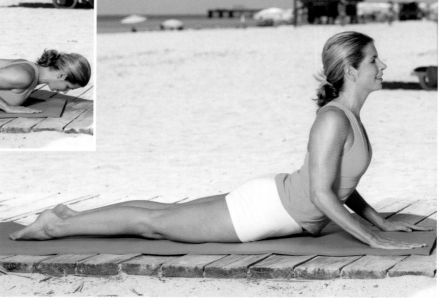

**STARTING POSITION:** Lie on your stomach with your legs straight, placing your hands directly under your shoulders, palms down. Elbows are close to your rib cage. Put some action in your butt cheeks and lift your belly button toward your spine.

## TIPS AND TRICKS

- Don't forget about the principles of extension: hip bones and pubic bone press into the mat; booty and hamstrings are engaged; armpits are dropped to your hips.

- Don't move your elbows to the sides of your chest; imagine a pencil between your arms and your rib cage, then squeeze it and shave your elbows past your rib cage to keep your elbows close to your body.

- Don't elevate your shoulders as you rock up and down; lower your shoulder blades down your back to stabilize your shoulders and open your chest.

**POSITION 1:** Inhale and slowly lift your chest off the mat, leading with your breastbone. Lift as high as you can, without feeling any pressure in your lower back. Exhale, lower to the mat, and quickly inhale up so you're rocking on your belly. Repeat 3 to 5 times.

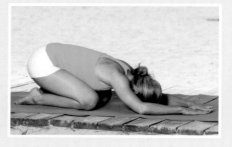

**POSITION 2:** Sit in a child's pose.

## THE PAYOFF:

Gives you a healthy belly and strong, fit back.

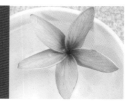

# Single Leg Kick

## REPLAY WEEKS ONE, TWO, THREE, FOUR, SIX

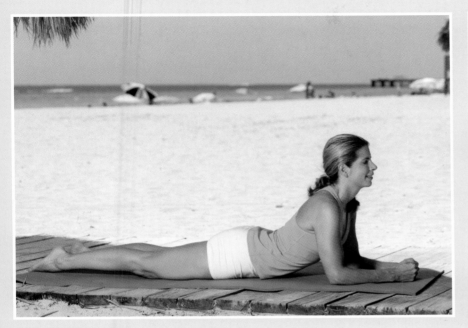

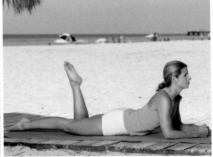

**POSITION 1:** Inhale, kick your right heel to your butt and then kick again.

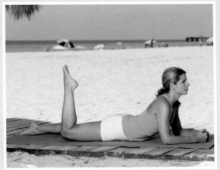

**POSITION 2:** Exhale, kick your right heel to your butt, and then kick again. Keep a steady rhythm going, both legs should be moving at the same time. Repeat 5 to 8 times.

**STARTING POSITION:** Lie on your stomach and lift your belly button toward your spine. Firm up your fanny and press your hip bones and pubic bone into the mat. Put your elbows directly under your shoulders and toward the belly to make an upside down "V," and press your elbows into the mat. Make two fists, and place your knuckles together.

### TIPS AND TRICKS

- Don't jiggle your booty; keep your pelvis stable and firm up your fanny.
- Don't round your shoulders; lift your head out of your shoulders as your breastbone lifts to the ceiling.
- Don't sag your belly; stay active to support your lower back. If you feel any lower back strain, put a pillow underneath your pelvis.

## THE PAYOFF:

Firms up your backside.

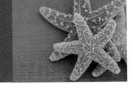

# Double Leg Kick

REPLAY WEEKS THREE, FOUR, SIX

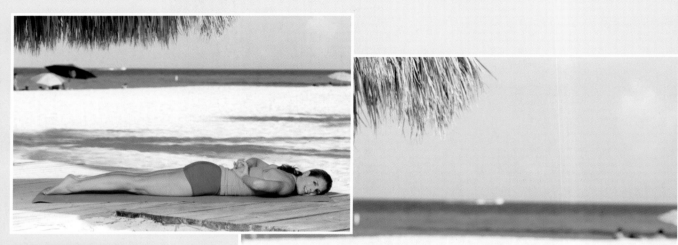

**STARTING POSITION:** Lie on your stomach with your legs straight, left cheek on the mat. Clasp your left hand around two fingers on your right hand, and position them in the middle of your back, elbows to the floor. You should feel a nice stretch across your back.

**TIPS AND TRICKS**

- Don't forget the principles of extension: press your hip bones and pubic bone into the mat; firm up your fanny and hamstrings; and don't flab your belly.

- Don't worry about the hand placement; just rest your hands on your lower back, palms up. When you lift into extension, just straighten your arms by your sides, palms down.

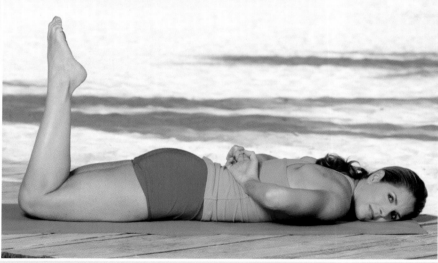

**POSITION 1:** Inhale to cue your body, then exhale to draw your heels to your bum; pulse three times to work your hamstrings. Don't lift your hip bones off the mat.

## THE PAYOFF:

Gives you a simply gorgeous, fit back.

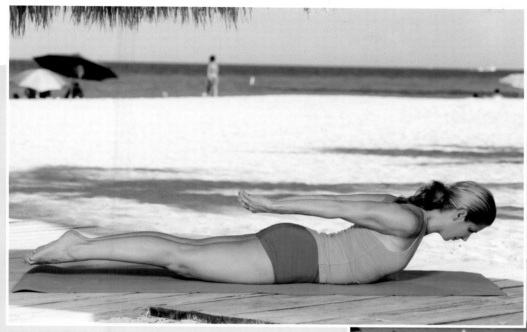

**POSITION 2:** Inhale into an extension of your spine while moving your arms down your back to lift your chest off the mat. The shoulder blades pull together to roll the shoulders back as you lift your clasped hands toward the ceiling to stretch your chest. Imagine shaving your arms down your back to draw your shoulders down.

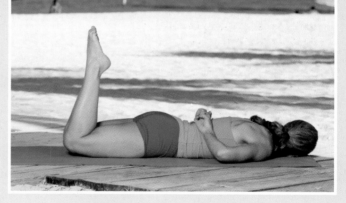

**POSITION 3:** Turn your cheek to the right, then exhale to draw your heels to your bum; pulse three times to work your hamstrings. Don't lift your hip bones off the mat. Do 3 to 5 reps, counting the right and left cheek as one rep.

# Neck Pull with Oblique Twist and 2-Pound Ball

REPLAY WEEK SIX

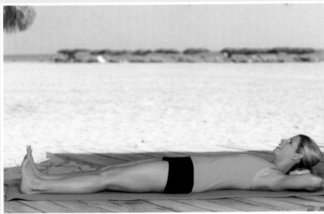

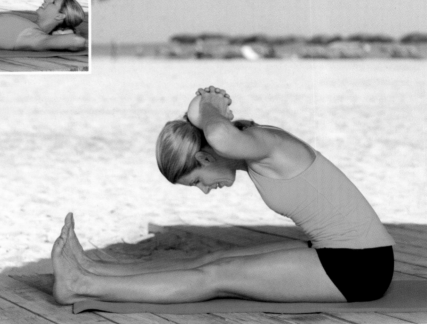

**STARTING POSITION:** Lie on your back with your legs straight, feet parallel and hip width apart. Hold a ball in your hands and clasp your hands behind your head so you can see your elbows out to the sides of your peripheral vision. Press your heels away from your hips, and be heavy in your heinie. Slide your shoulder blades down your back.

## TIPS AND TRICKS

- Don't hide your face as you roll up; your elbows are in your peripheral vision or lengthened out to the sides.

- Don't plop down; press your heels away from your hips as you roll down and scoop!

- Don't strain your lower back; if you feel a twinge in your lower back, drop the ball and complete the steps.

- Don't just twist; move from your rib cage to get the added oblique work.

**POSITION 1:** Inhale to lift your head off the mat to curl your chin to your chest to initiate peeling your spine off the mat, keep your neck long. Exhale to round over, nose to your belly button.

## THE PAYOFF:

Uncovers strong, sexy, flat abs.

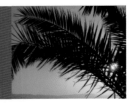

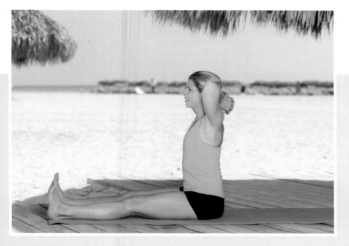

**POSITION 2:** Inhale to stack your vertebrae as you uncurl your spine, lifting your head to the ceiling until you're sitting out of your hips.

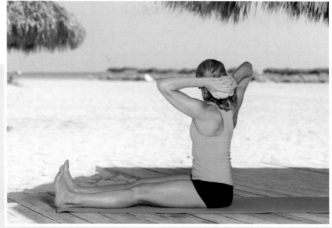

**POSITION 3:** Exhale to twist your torso to the right, leading with your bottom ribs.

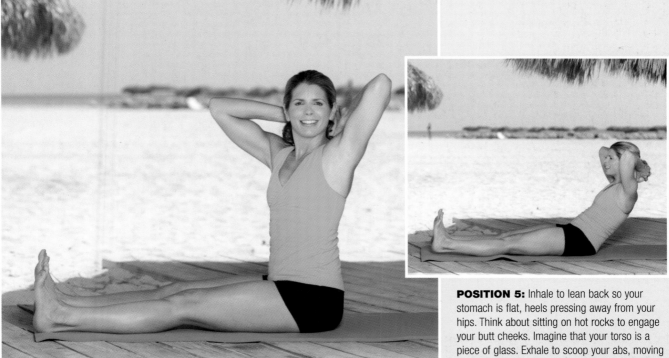

**POSITION 4:** Inhale to the center and then exhale to twist your torso to the left.

**POSITION 5:** Inhale to lean back so your stomach is flat, heels pressing away from your hips. Think about sitting on hot rocks to engage your butt cheeks. Imagine that your torso is a piece of glass. Exhale to scoop your abs, moving your pubic bone to the ceiling, and roll down vertebra by vertebra to the mat. Repeat 3 to 5 times.

# Shoulder Bridge with One Leg

REPLAY WEEKS THREE, FOUR, SIX

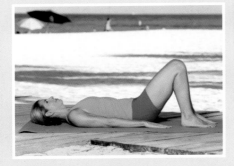

**STARTING POSITION:** Lie on your back with your arms straight by your sides and place your feet about hip width apart. Inhale to cue your body.

## TIPS AND TRICKS

- Don't sag in your booty; keep your hips even and maintain a neutral position to build your core strength.
- Use your abs; stay solid from your breastbone to your pubic bone even as you lift your leg, the tendency is for one hip to droop.

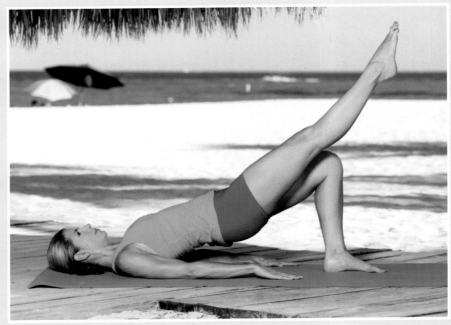

**POSITION 1:** Exhale to scoop your abs and lift your spine off the mat vertebra by vertebra. Once you're stable, lift your right leg and count to 5 to challenge your core even more! Inhale to roll down, vertebra by vertebra.

## THE PAYOFF:

Perks up your booty and creates a strong core.

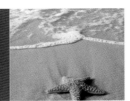

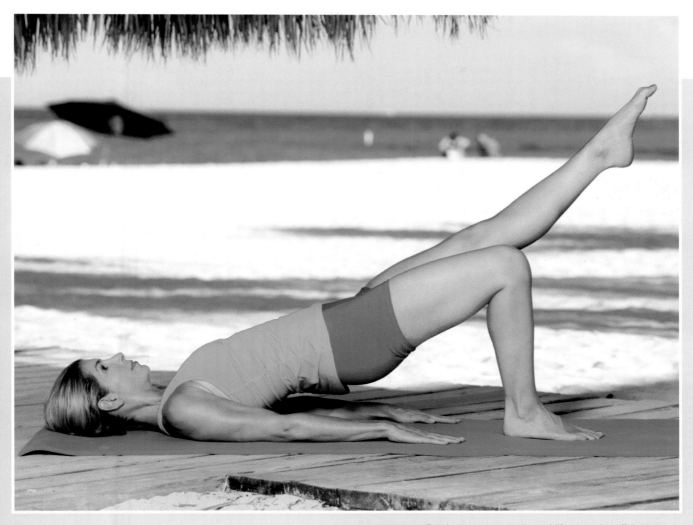

**POSITION 2:** Exhale to scoop your abs and lift your spine off the mat vertebra by vertebra. Lift your left leg and count to 5 to challenge your core even more! Inhale to roll down, vertebra by vertebra, as if you were lying in sand. Imagine a sling is hanging from the ceiling to hoist your hips and prevent your bottom from sinking into the mat. Repeat 3 to 5 times.

# Teaser Twist with 2-Pound Ball

REPLAY WEEK SIX

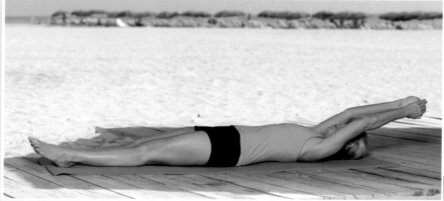

**STARTING POSITION:** Lie on your back with your legs straight and your arms straight over your head. Hold the ball in your hands.

### TIPS AND TRICKS

- Don't strain in your lower back.
- Don't plop down; scoop and uncurl your spine to lower to the mat with control.
- If this exercise is too hard with the ball, drop it and follow the same exact steps.

**POSITION 1:** At the same time, inhale to lift your arms to your legs into a "V," your fingertips reaching for your toes. Scoop, scoop, scoop to build strength and protect your back

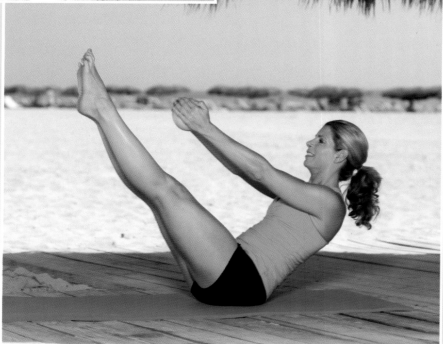

## THE PAYOFF:

Moves you from so-so to stunning abs.

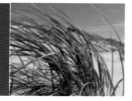

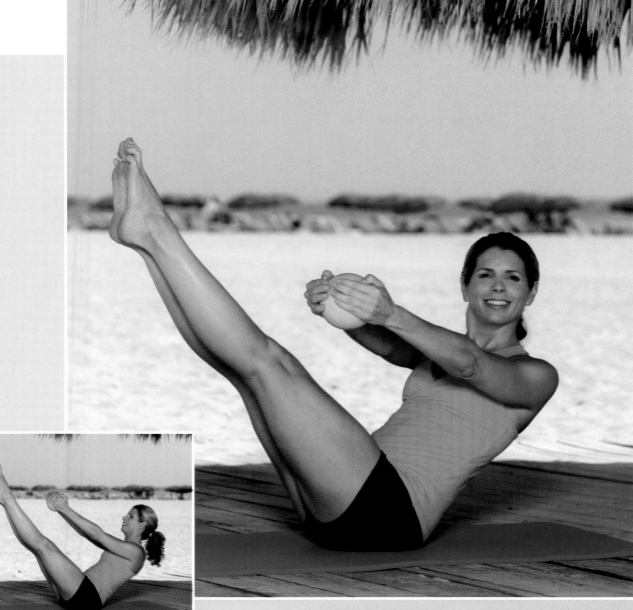

**POSITION 3:** Exhale to twist your torso to the left. Inhale to center, and exhale to roll down slowly to the mat. Repeat 3 to 5 times.

**POSITION 2:** Exhale to twist your torso to the right, and inhale back to the center.

# The Seal

REPLAY WEEKS ONE, TWO, THREE, FOUR, SIX

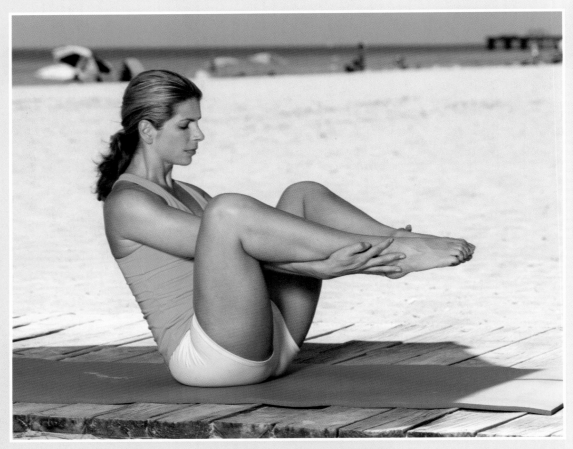

**STARTING POSITION:** Sit at the edge of the mat and slide your heels to your booty. Drive into your legs and wrap your arms under and around so your hands end up on the outside of your ankles. Look at your belly as you drop your chin to your chest, rounding your spine.

**TIPS AND TRICKS**

- Engage your inner thighs when you clap your heels.
- Don't roll onto your head or neck; it's the upper back and shoulders that absorb the weight of your body.

## THE PAYOFF:

Leads to a flexible, fit spine.

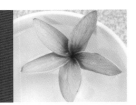

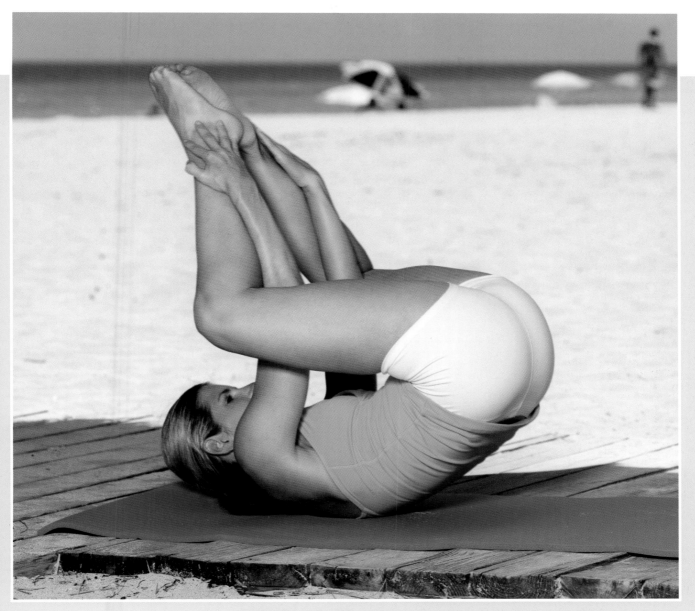

**POSITION 1:** Move your pubic bone to the ceiling while scooping your abs. Hold this scoop, then lift your feet off the mat. Engage your abs to maintain your pelvic stability, and clap your heels and bark like a seal. (Why not? It's free and fun.) Inhale to roll back to your upper back, only. Exhale to roll up. Pause, clap your heels 3 times, and roll again, scooping your belly the whole time to find your balance and clap your heels together. Repeat 8 to 10 times.

# SUNDAY: BEING LAZY!

You and everyone else will notice how hot your body looks! Don't lose momentum as you take this day off. Instead, add a few more healthy eating habits that will get you bikini ready:

- **Snack on berries:** Get brain-healthy benefits and antioxidants with a smoothie made with blueberries, strawberries, or blackberries, which are so good for a healthy bikini body.

- **Eat more chocolate:** Dark chocolate is full of antioxidants. It satisfies your sweet craving yet helps you maintain your bikini bod, if you don't overdo it!

Okay girls, six weeks ago, you were snug in your sweaters. Now, you can taste those umbrella drinks and feel the sand between your toes. You're going to make your own waves and turn heads along the way. Keep it up, and you'll bare your best bikini body all summer long.

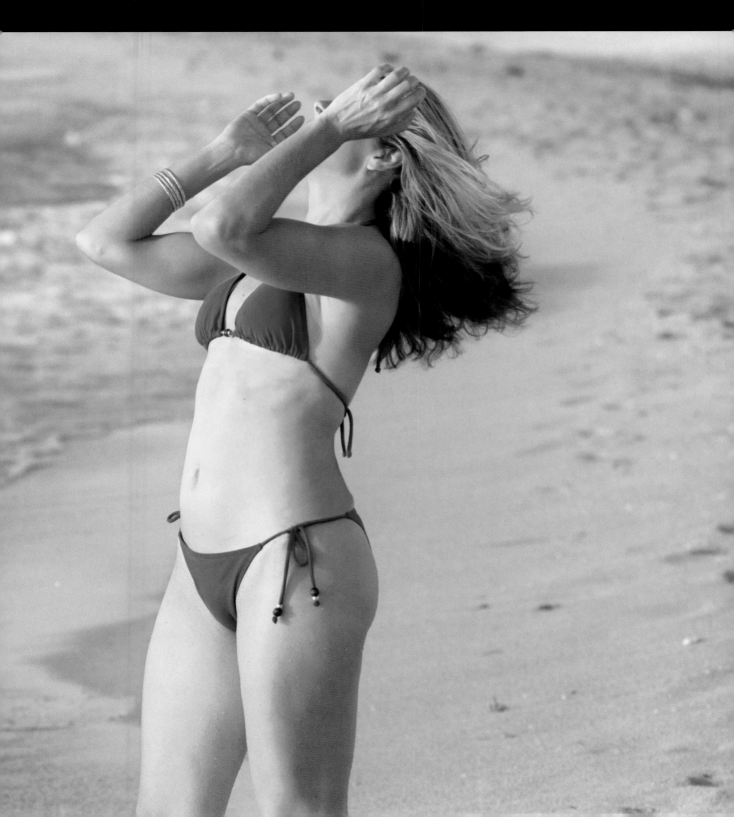

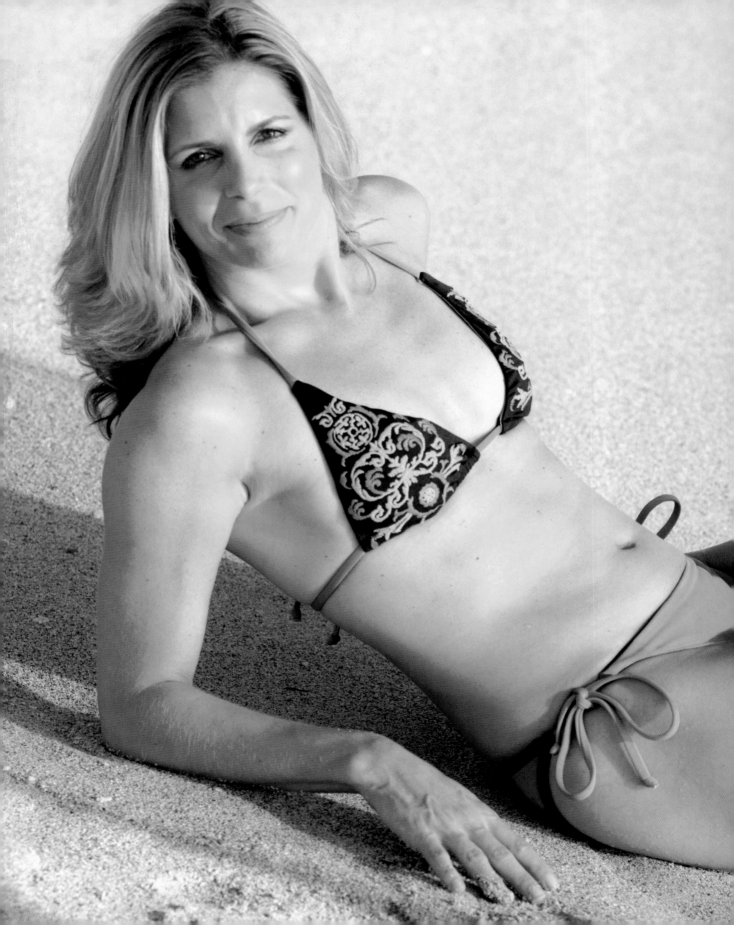

## GET YOUR BEST BIKINI SELF AND BOOTY

As a result of all your hard work, you're off to your best bikini body. You should have seen some exciting body changes: leaner legs, firmer bum, and those abs to die for. Now, it's time to get fabulous and fearless in your bikini. You're in better shape, so you can burn lots more calories. This week, you'll work a bit harder to scorch calories and put some finishing touches on your bottom line. Finish strong and then watch your body become beach-worthy!

**MONDAY**        Becoming Fabulous with Boot-Camp-Strength Intervals

**TUESDAY**       Getting Bikini Lean with Steady-State Cardio

**WEDNESDAY**  Busting Your Booty with Pilates

**THURSDAY**     Becoming Fabulous with Boot-Camp-Strength Intervals

**FRIDAY**          Getting Bikini Lean with Steady-State Cardio

**SATURDAY**     Busting Your Booty with Pilates

**SUNDAY**         Celebrating You!

# week six

## WORKOUT PROGRAM AT A GLANCE

M T W T

| MONDAY | TUESDAY | WEDNESDAY | THURSDAY |
|---|---|---|---|
| **Becoming Fabulous with Boot-Camp-Strength Intervals** | **Getting Bikini Lean with Steady-State Cardio** | **Busting Your Booty with Pilates** | **Becoming Fabulous with Boot-Camp-Strength Intervals** |
| **SET 1**<br><br>Jump Curtsy<br><br>Ball Bridge with Chest Press<br><br>Single Leg Triceps Extension<br><br>**SET 2**<br><br>Plyo-Lunge<br><br>Ball Bridge with Reverse Fly<br><br>Plank on Ball<br><br>**SET 3**<br><br>Jump Squat on Step<br><br>Single Leg Biceps Curl<br><br>Push-up and Reverse Ab Curl Combination | Warm up for 3 minutes at an easy pace (level 4 or 5 on the intensity scale discussed in the introduction of this book), and then move your body to a breathless, sweaty pace for 45 minutes (level 7), before doing a 2-minute cool/down at level 3 or 4 again. | **After doing the Pilates Abs in week five, do the following Pilates exercises today:**<br><br>Side Kick Front and Push Back with 2-Pound Ball<br><br>Push Back with Outer Thigh Lift Combo with 2-Pound Ball<br><br>Leg Circle with 2-Pound Ball<br><br>Hot Potato with 2-Pound Ball<br><br>Clam with 2-Pound Ball<br><br>Booty Buster on Big Ball<br><br>Big Ball Beats on Belly<br><br>Froggy with Big Ball<br><br>Inner Thigh Squeeze with Big Ball | **SET 1**<br><br>Jump Curtsy<br><br>Ball Bridge with Chest Press<br><br>Single Leg Triceps Extension<br><br>**SET 2**<br><br>Plyo-Lunge<br><br>Ball Bridge with Reverse Fly<br><br>Plank on Ball<br><br>**SET 3**<br><br>Jump Squat on Step<br><br>Single Leg Biceps Curl<br><br>Push-up and Reverse Ab Curl Combination |

| F | S | S |
|---|---|---|
| **FRIDAY** | **SATURDAY** | **SUNDAY** |
| Getting Bikini Lean with Steady-State Cardio | Busting Your Booty with Pilates | Celebrating You! |

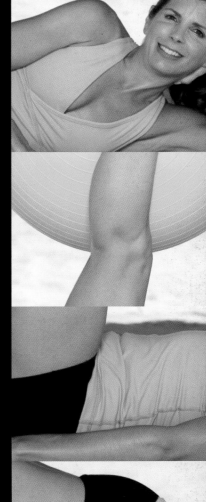

**FRIDAY**

Warm up for 3 minutes at an easy pace (level 4 or 5 on the intensity scale discussed in the introduction of this book), and then move your body to a breathless, sweaty pace for 45 minutes (level 7), before doing a 2-minute cool/down at level 3 or 4 again.

**SATURDAY**

**After doing the Pilates Abs in week five, do the following Pilates exercises today:**

Side Kick Front and Push Back with 2-Pound Ball

Push Back with Outer Thigh Lift Combo with 2-Pound Ball

Leg Circle with 2-Pound Ball

Hot Potato with 2-Pound Ball

Clam with 2-Pound Ball

Booty Buster on Big Ball

Big Ball Beats on Belly

Froggy with Big Ball

Inner Thigh Squeeze with Big Ball

**SUNDAY**

OFF

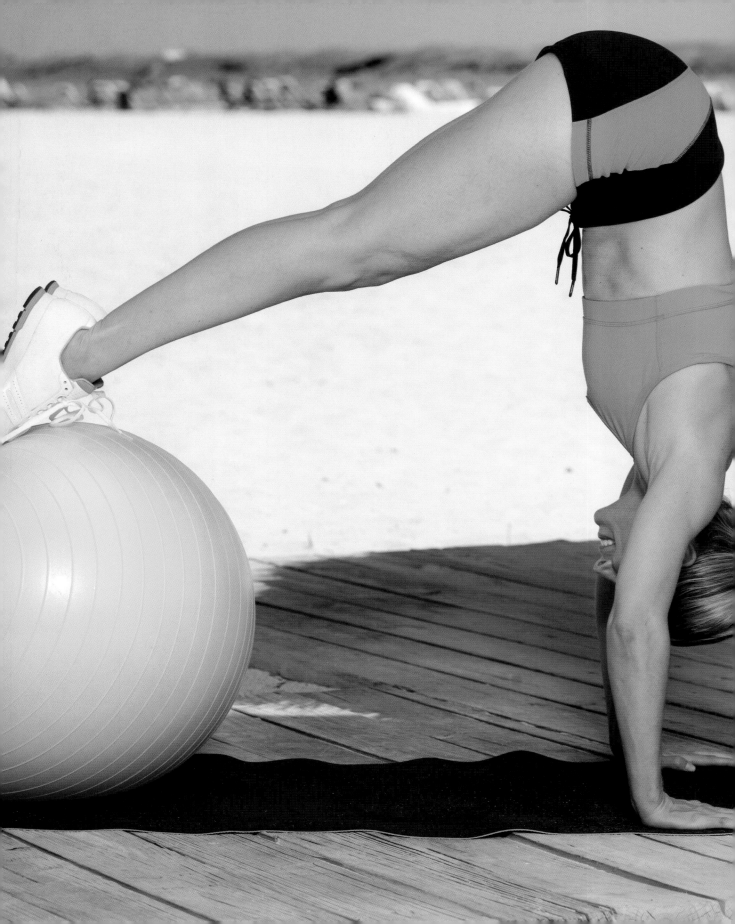

# MONDAY: BECOMING FABULOUS WITH BOOT-CAMP-STRENGTH INTERVALS

Your firm and fabulous strategy is all about taking it up a bit to burn fat and build muscles. Because you're already feeling fit, these exercises push you to the next level. Remember that, to burn mega calories, you'll do both cardio and strength training in this week's boot camp workouts. Your goal is to move from exercise to exercise with no more than 30 seconds of rest, and alternate between heavy breathing and choppy talk to demanding yet doable recovery (see the introduction for more on determining your intensity levels). You'll need an 8- or 10-pound (4 to 5 kg) set of dumbbells for your arms, a 15- or 20-pound set of dumbbells for your legs, plus a stability ball. Do these two 45-minute to 1-hour boot camp workouts today and on Thursday.

To do this boot camp workout you'll do 15 to 20 reps of each exercise in a set, and then repeat the set twice more. For example, complete 15 to 20 slow and controlled reps of each exercise in Set 1: Jump Curtsy, Ball Bridge with Chest Press, and Single Leg Triceps Extension. Repeat that set twice more before moving on to Set 2, and then finish with Set 3. Total time should be about 45 minutes to 1 hour. If you're not clear on what a set or a rep is, flip to the introduction to this book. And don't forget to warm up on the treadmill for 5 minutes at 3.5 mph (5.5 kph).

**SET 1**

Jump Curtsy

Ball Bridge with Chest Press

Single Leg Triceps Extension

**SET 2**

Plyo-Lunge

Ball Bridge with Reverse Fly

Plank on Ball

**SET 3**

Jump Squat on Step

Single Leg Biceps Curl

Push-up and Reverse Ab Curl Combination

# Jump Curtsy

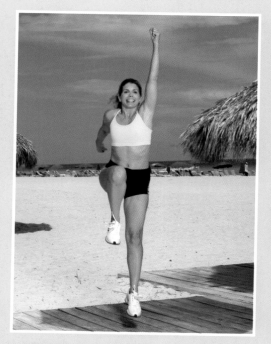

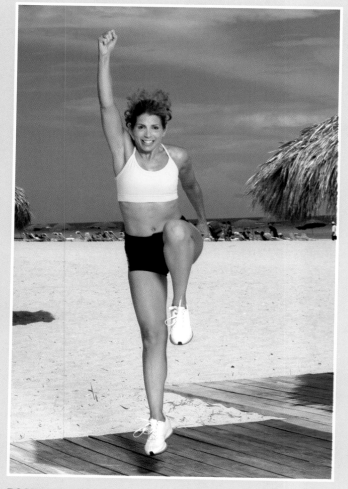

**STARTING POSITION:** Stand hip width apart with your hands by your sides. Jump up, lifting your right knee and left arm to the ceiling.

**TIPS AND TRICKS**

- Don't just lift your knee; explode, using your arm to propel you higher into the air.
- Don't land like an elephant; come down softly as you change legs: it's a step, kick ball change, to get to the other side.

**POSITION 1:** When you land, take two steps back or do a step-kick ball change and then jump with the left leg (left knee and right arms lift). This is one rep. Do 15 to 20 reps.

## THE PAYOFF:

Scorches calories and take inches off your legs.

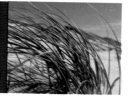

# Ball Bridge with Chest Press

REPLAY WEEK FIVE

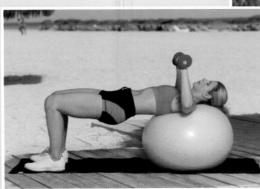

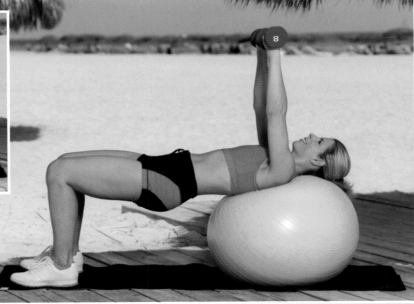

**STARTING POSITION:** Hold an 8- to 10-pound (4 to 5 kg) dumbbell in each hand, sit on the center of your ball, and walk down until your upper back is on the ball. While in the bridge position, bend your elbows out to the sides of your shoulders, knuckles up.

## TIPS AND TRICKS

- Don't sag in your booty; lift from your backside.
- Don't haphazardly lift or lower your arms; use your core and control each rep.

**POSITION 1:** In a count of 4, press your arms to the ceiling, then slowly lower your arms to the ball.

## THE PAYOFF:

Develops sexy curves in your chest and shoulders.

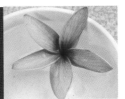

# Single Leg Triceps Extension

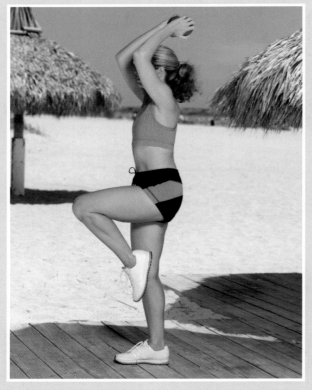

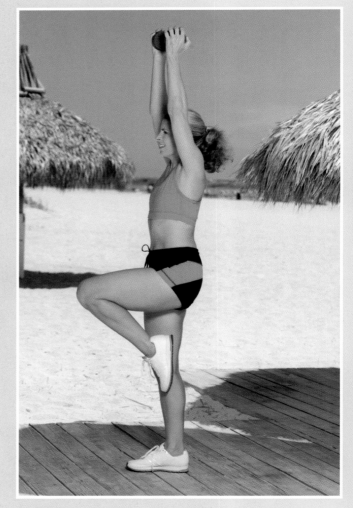

**STARTING POSITION:** Stand with feet hip width apart and hold an 8- to 10-pound (4 to 5 kg) dumbbell in both hands. Lift your arms over your head so your elbows bend forward as the weight drops behind your head at about a 90-degree angle. Stand tall and lift your left knee to hip height.

**TIPS AND TRICKS**

- Don't bulge your abs; engage your core muscles to help you balance, especially as you lower and lift the weight to the ceiling.
- Don't look down; lengthen from the top of your head and gaze at a spot on the wall to help you balance.
- Don't swing your elbows; keep them stable to fully work your triceps.

**POSITION 1:** In a count of 4, lift the dumbbell to the ceiling, then slowly lower the dumbbell. Do 10 reps on your left leg, and then 10 reps on your right.

# THE PAYOFF:

Leads to incredibly sexy arms.

# Plyo-Lunge

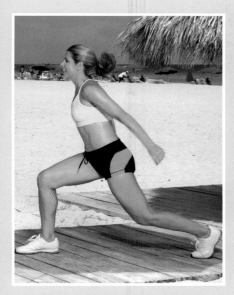

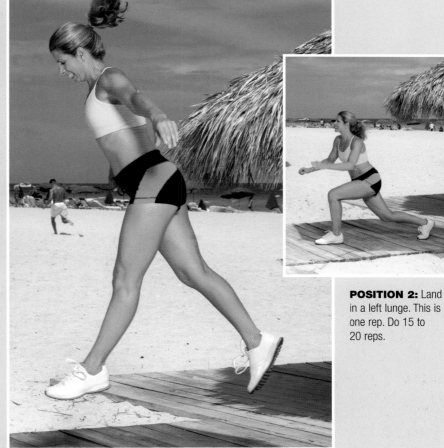

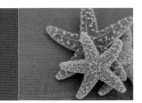

**STARTING POSITION:** In a lunge position with your right leg forward and your arms out in front of you.

### TIPS AND TRICKS

- Don't lean forward too much; use your arms to help you balance.

- Don't let your knee move past your second and third toes; the majority of your body weight is in the lunge leg.

- Remember your core; exhale to give you lots of power and help keep you steady.

**POSITION 1:** Jump up (explode) as high as you can go and switch legs.

**POSITION 2:** Land in a left lunge. This is one rep. Do 15 to 20 reps.

## THE PAYOFF:

Burns calories and leads to strong legs and a firm butt.

# Ball Bridge with Reverse Fly

REPLAY WEEK FIVE

**STARTING POSITION:** Sit on the center of your ball with your knees touching, feet parallel and firmly grounded to the floor. Hold an 8- to 10-pound (4 to 5 kg) dumbbell in each hand and bend forward at the waist until your chest just about touches your thighs. Lift your breastbone slightly to help maintain a stable spine while your arms dangle by your ankles, palms down. Gaze at the floor.

### TIPS AND TRICKS

- Don't round your spine; lift from your breastbone to help keep your spine straight.

- Don't swing your arms; imagine cracking a walnut between your shoulder blades as your arms move behind you to engage a variety of upper back muscles, including your rhomboids.

- If you can't move with control, switch to a lighter weight or don't use dumbbells at all. Your rear or posterior deltoid is usually the weakest of all your shoulder muscles, so start out with light weights.

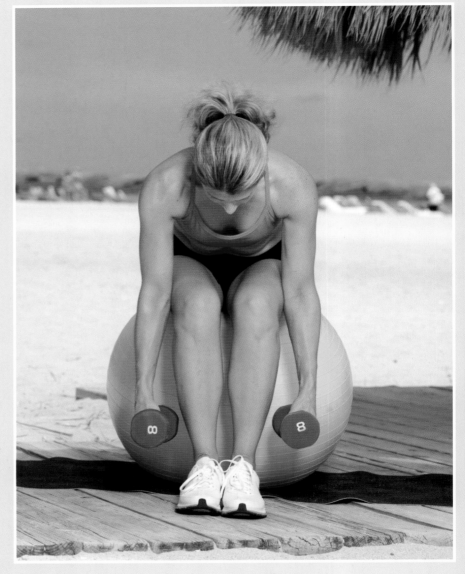

## THE PAYOFF:

Makes for a sexy, sculpted back and shoulders.

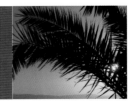

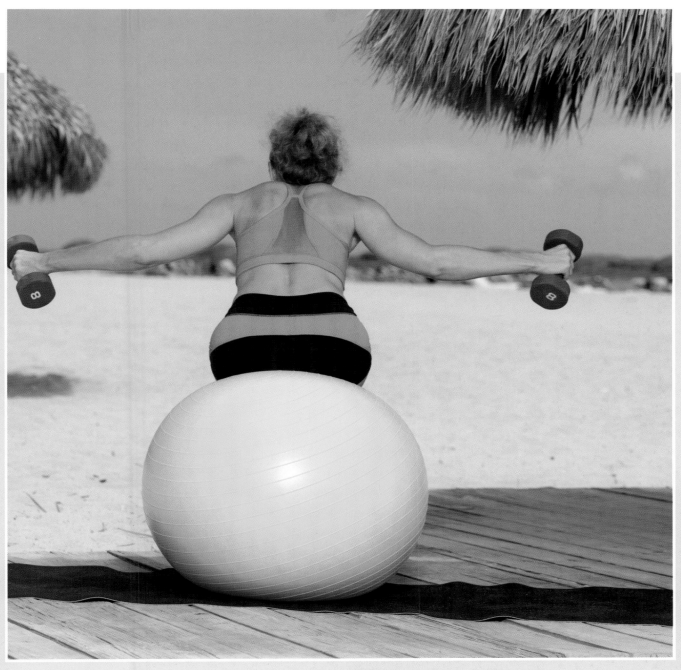

**POSITION 1:** In a count of 4, lift your arms up and out to the sides, about shoulder height, then slowly lower your arms. Do 15 to 20 reps.

# Plank on Ball

REPLAY WEEK FIVE

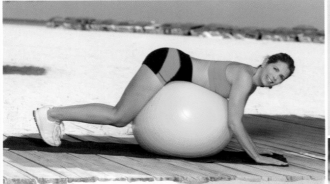

**STARTING POSITION:** Kneel in front of your ball and drape your abdomen and hips over the ball. Place your hands on the floor in front of the ball.

**TIPS AND TRICKS**

- Use your legs; contract between your inner thighs for extra power—ladies, it works!

- Don't do this exercise if you have a shoulder or neck injury.

- Don't open your arms too wide; align your wrists directly under your shoulders while your shoulder blades slide down your back to create shoulder stability and work your upper back muscles. To alleviate wrist pain, consider using a pair of dumbbell weights to elevate your wrists in a neutral position.

- Don't sag your belly; if you feel pressure in your lower back, make sure your hips are not below the ball, and lift your belly button to the sky with every deep exhale.

- Don't drop your head; lengthen from the top of your head and gaze at the floor.

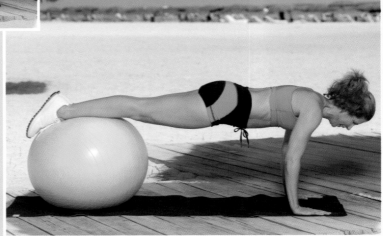

**POSITION 1:** Walk your hands out until the ball rolls toward your shins. Once you're stable, hold for 30 seconds as your body remains solid and straight, your back perfectly straight, like steel. Squeeze your thighs for inner thigh power. Focus on your exhale to engage your core and to keep you steady on the ball.

## THE PAYOFF:

Takes inches off all over and reveals a sexy core.

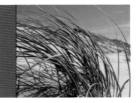

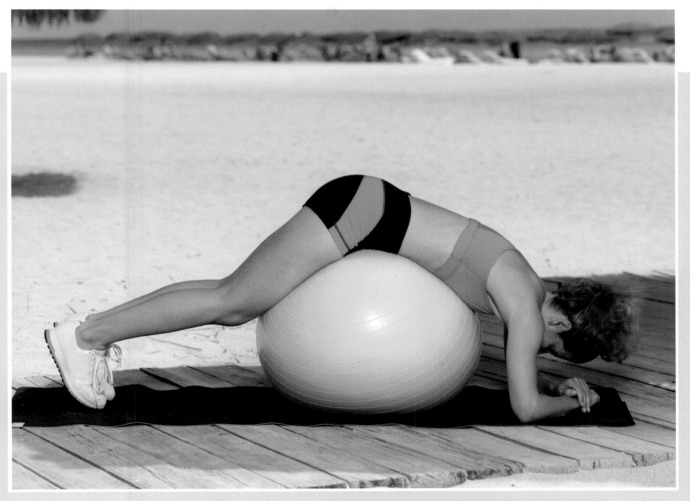

**POSITION 2:** Drape your body over the ball to stretch your lower back.

## ⭐ CORE COMPLETE

Plank is the ultimate multi muscle move: you can do a variety of levels if you're not ready for this advanced position. Putting the ball under your belly is the easiest; putting the ball under your thighs is a little harder; and putting the ball under your shins or ankles is the most difficult because gravity challenges your entire torso, creating a big core workout!

# Jump Squat on Step

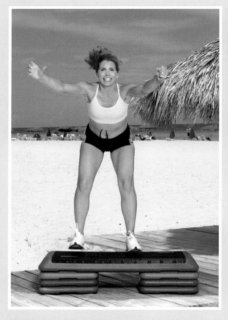

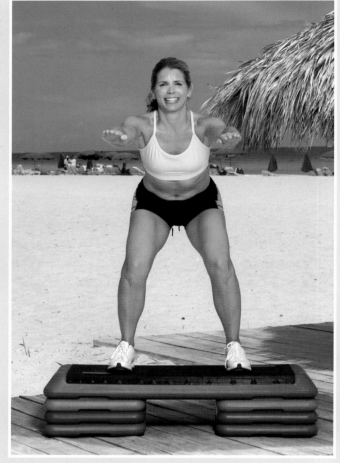

**STARTING POSITION:** Stand behind your step (about 5 or 6 rises) and straighten your arms by your sides and jump up and land in a squat.

**TIPS AND TRICKS**

- Don't drop your chest; stay lifted and long in your spine.
- Use your arms to help you explode; remember, you're going for power moves to bring your heart rate up.

**POSITION 1:** Land softly with the majority of body weight in your heels, with both knees parallel to the step, with your arms out in front. Walk down. Do 15 to 20 reps.

## THE PAYOFF:

Burns away calories and firms up your backside.

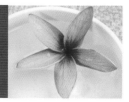

# Single Leg Biceps Curl

REPLAY WEEK FIVE

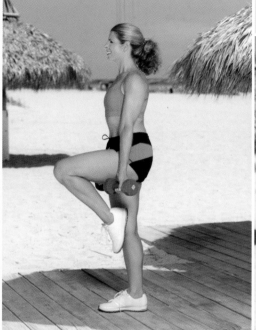

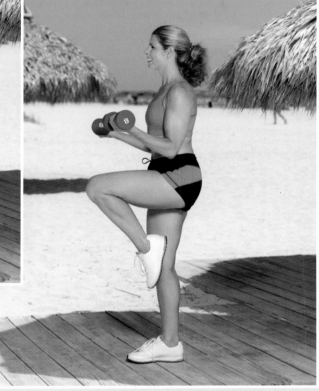

**STARTING POSITION:** Stand hip width apart and hold an 8- to 10-pound (4 to 5 kg) dumbbell in each hand. At the same time, lift your left knee hip-height and lower your arms by your sides. Lengthen from the top of your head to maintain a straight spine.

## TIPS AND TRICKS

- Engage your core muscles to help you balance as you lift the weights.
- Don't look down; find a spot on the wall and gaze at it to help you balance.
- Don't swing your elbows as you curl; use smooth and controlled movements.

**POSITION 1:** In a count of 4, curl the dumbbells to your chest, then slowly lower them. Do 10 reps on the left leg, then 10 reps on the right.

## THE PAYOFF:

Sculpts sexy, strong arms.

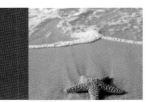

# Push-up and Reverse Ab Curl Combination

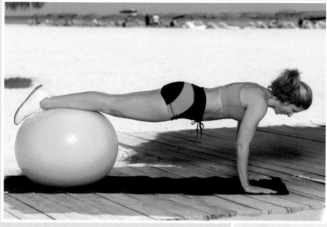

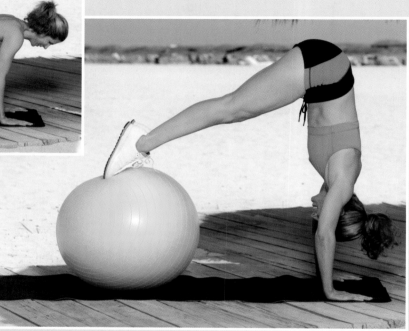

**STARTING POSITION:** Kneel in front of your ball and round your chest, abdomen, and hips over it. Place your hands on the floor in front of the ball. Walk your hands out until you are in a plank position, with your feet on the ball and your body forming a straight line. Make sure your hands are directly under your shoulders. Inhale to a plank position.

**TIPS AND TRICKS**

- Breathe! Your exhale will force your abs into action and help lift your hips and support your lower back.

- Don't drop your head; look at the floor while lengthening from the top of your head so it makes a straight line with your body.

**POSITION 1:** Exhale to lift your hips to the sky so that your body forms an upside-down "V."

## THE PAYOFF:

Leads to oodles of allover tone and sexy, flat abs.

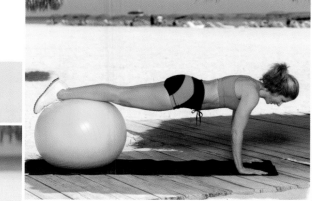

**POSITION 2:** Inhale to a plank position.

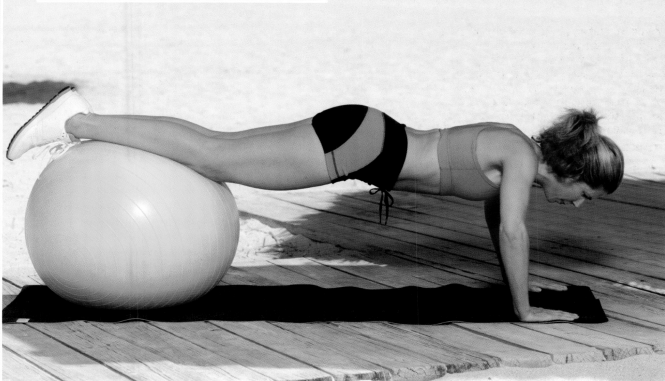

**POSITION 3:** Exhale as you bend your elbows out to the sides, lowering your body to the floor to do a push-up. Do 15 to 20 reps.

# TUESDAY: GETTING BIKINI LEAN WITH STEADY-STATE CARDIO

This week, you'll do a cardio circuit, blending several machines, such as 15 minutes on the treadmill, 15 minutes on the stair stepper, and 20 minutes on the elliptical trainer, plus a few minutes to warm up and cool down, totaling a 50- to 55-minute cardio session. Mix and match as you see fit, using a stationary bike, treadmill, stair stepper, elliptical trainer, or any other cardio machine you have access to. If you don't have a gym membership, take a 50- to 55-minute run or power walk outside. Warm up for 3 minutes at an easy pace (level 3 or 4 on the intensity scale discussed in the introduction of this book), and then move your body to a breathless, sweaty pace for 45 minutes (level 7), before doing a 2 minute cool down at level 3 or 4 again.

# WEDNESDAY: BUSTING YOUR BOOTY WITH PILATES

Okay, you know what to do, add these oh-so-fab exercises to your Pilates workout from week five, right after you finish with The Seal exercise. Gather up some fun toys such as a big ball and two 2-pound (1 kg) balls and your butt will thank you! As always, follow the instructions and do 10 to 20 reps of each exercise (more like 20, please), unless I state otherwise. Start out on the right leg, and then after you finish the Inner Thigh Squeeze exercise, repeat all the exercises on the left leg.

Check out these booty-busting exercises you'll be doing today:

- Side Kick Front and Push Back with 2-Pound Ball
- Push Back with Outer Thigh Lift Combo with 2-Pound Ball
- Leg Circle with 2-Pound Ball
- Hot Potato with 2-Pound Ball
- Clam with 2-Pound Ball
- Booty Buster on Big Ball
- Big Ball Beats on Belly
- Froggy with Big Ball
- Inner Thigh Squeeze with Big Ball

# Side Kick Front and Push Back with 2-Pound Ball

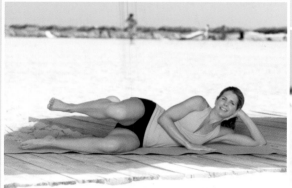

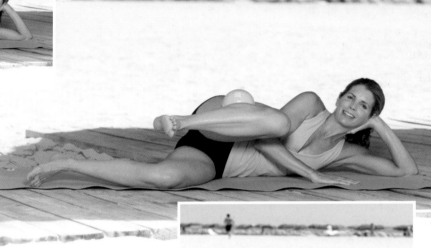

**STARTING POSITION:** Lie on your left side with your knees bent in front of you so your ankles, knees, and hip bones are stacked on top of one another. Prop your head up with your left arm and then place your right arm, palm down, on the mat in front of your torso; relax your shoulders. Put a 2-pound (1 kg) ball behind your right knee and lift your top leg to hip height so it's parallel to the floor.

### TIPS AND TRICKS

- Don't lower your foot; keep your foot in alignment with your hip to get that yummy outer thigh work.

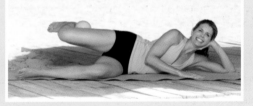

**POSITION 1:** Inhale to move your leg forward.

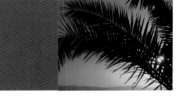

**POSITION 2:** Exhale to move your leg back, pushing with your heel to firm up your fanny.

## THE PAYOFF:

Tightens, tones, and de-dimples your hips.

# Push Back with Outer Thigh Lift Combo with 2-Pound Ball

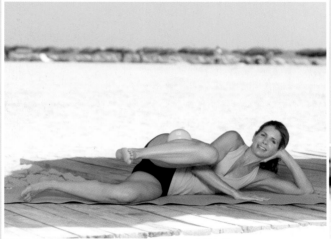

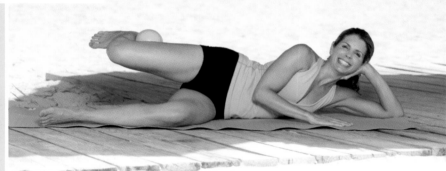

**STARTING POSITION:** Lie on your left side with your knees bent in front of you so your ankles, knees, and hip bones are stacked on top of one another. Prop your head up with your left arm and then place your right arm, palm down, on the mat in front of your torso; relax your shoulders. Put a 2-pound (1 kg) ball behind your right knee. Lift your top leg to hip height so it's parallel to the floor and then inhale to move your leg forward.

## TIPS AND TRICKS

- Don't drop your knee; keep it hip height to get the yummy outer thigh work.

- Don't drop your heel; keep it hip height to work your booty.

**POSITION 1:** Exhale to move the leg behind you, pushing with the heel of your foot firm up your fanny.

## THE PAYOFF:

Allows you to say bye-bye to dimples.

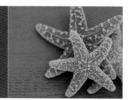

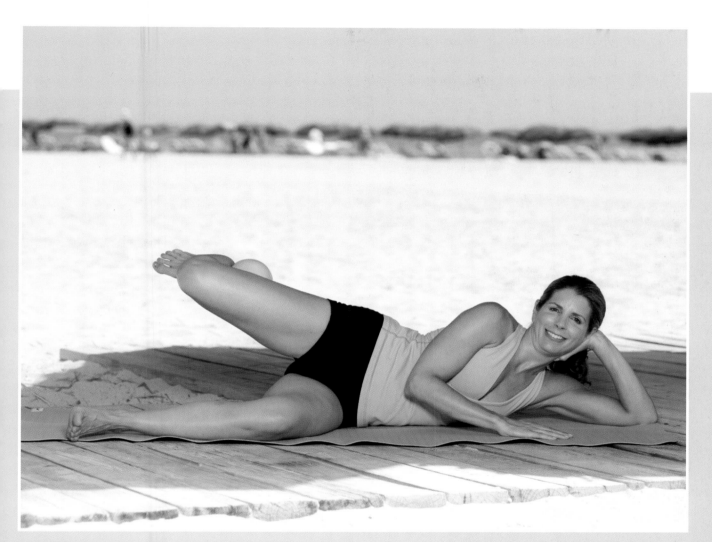

**POSITION 2:** After pushing your heel back to work your butt, lift your leg
to the ceiling to work your outer thigh.

# Leg Circle with 2-Pound Ball

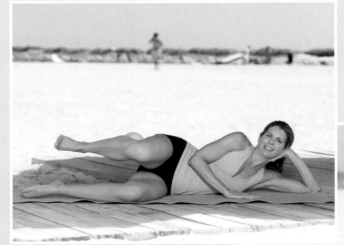

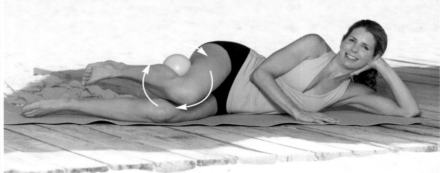

**STARTING POSITION:** Lie on your left side with your knees bent in front of you so your ankles, knees, and hip bones are stacked on top of one another. Prop your head up with your left arm and then place your right arm, palm down, on the mat in front of your torso; relax your shoulders. Put the 2-pound (1 kg) ball behind your left knee and lift your top leg to hip height so it's parallel to the floor.

## TIPS AND TRICKS

- Don't drop your knee as you circle; your leg should always stay hip height to get the outer thigh work.

- Remember to keep your circles small to completely de-dimple your thighs.

**POSITION 1:** Circle the leg in front; these are tiny circles.

## THE PAYOFF:

Shrinks your thighs and scorches dimples.

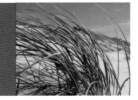

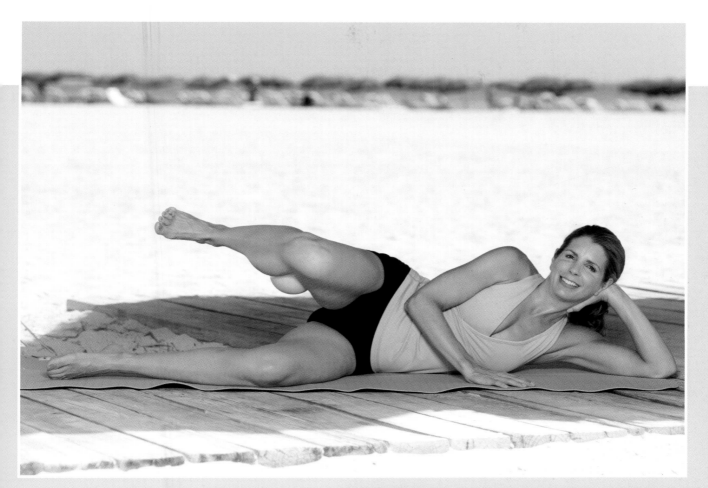

**POSITION 2:** Make sure your leg is high enough that your outer thigh is working. After 20 circles, reverse directions and do 20 more. Breathe normally.

# Hot Potato with 2-Pound Ball

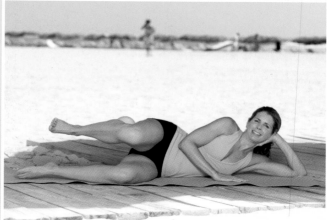

**STARTING POSITION:** Lie on your left side with your knees bent in front of you so your ankles, knees, and hip bones are stacked on top of one another. Prop your head up with your left arm and then place your right arm, palm down, on the mat in front of your torso; relax your shoulders. Put the 2-pound (1 kg) ball behind your left knee and lift your top leg to hip height so it's parallel to the floor.

**TIPS AND TRICKS**

- Don't move your knee; keep it at an angle to the floor to get the yummy outer thigh work.
- Don't drop your heel; keep it high to work your booty.

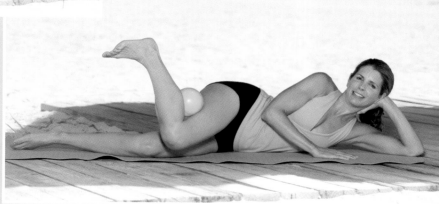

**POSITION 1:** Inhale to turn your knee to the ground and tap it to the mat in front of your thigh.

## THE PAYOFF:

Takes serious inches off your thighs and scorches your butt.

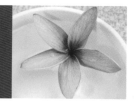

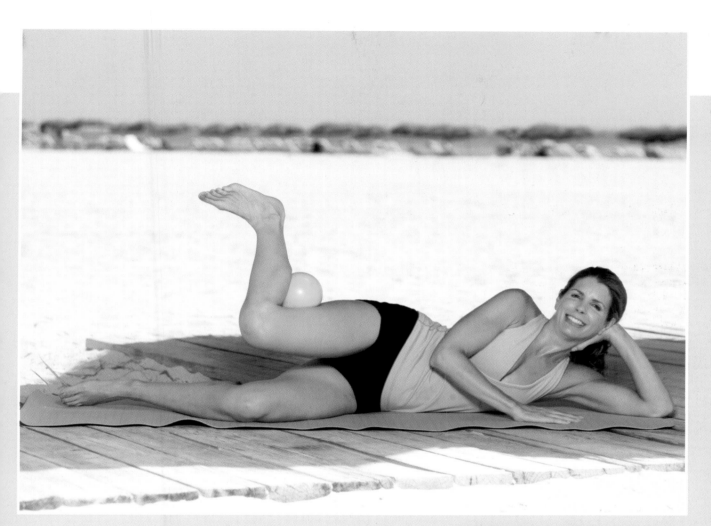

**POSITION 3:** Exhale to lift your heel to the ceiling and feel your booty work.

# Clam with 2-Pound Ball

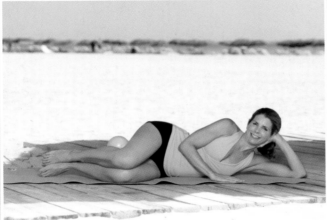

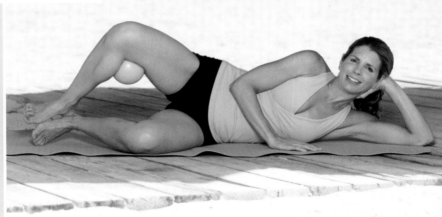

**STARTING POSITION:** Lie on your left side with your knees bent in front of you so your ankles, knees, and hip bones are stacked on top of one another. Prop your head up with your left arm and then place your right arm, palm down, on the mat in front of your torso; relax your shoulders. Put a 2-pound (1 kg) ball behind your right knee.

## TIPS AND TRICKS

- Don't separate your heels; open your knees just high enough to feel the outer thigh work.

**POSITION 1:** Inhale to lift your knee to the ceiling without lifting your heel. Your heels are glued together and you won't be able to lift your knee very high.

## THE PAYOFF:

Fights cellulite and underbutt.

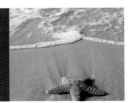

# Booty Buster on Big Ball

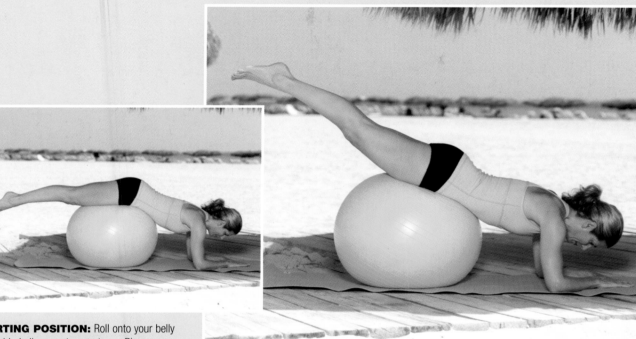

**STARTING POSITION:** Roll onto your belly so the big ball supports your torso. Place your elbows on the floor in front of the ball. Gaze at the floor.

## TIPS AND TRICKS

- Don't sag your belly; lift your belly button to the sky to give your lower back support.
- Don't forget to firm up your fanny; put a thousand dollar bill between your butt cheeks —well, at least imagine it!

**POSITION 1:** Lift both legs up off the ball, lifting from your fanny and squeezing your inner thighs. If you need a rest, drape yourself over the ball after you're done and just breathe. It's a yummy lower back stretch.

## THE PAYOFF:

Tightens your tushie, one dimple at a time.

# Big Ball Beats on Belly

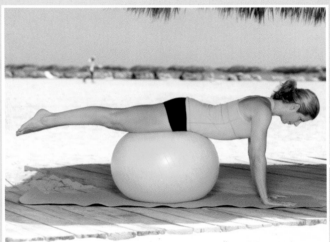

**STARTING POSITION:** Roll onto your hips so the ball supports your torso. Place your hands on the floor in front of the ball. Gaze at the floor. Lift your legs, engaging your glutes, heels together.

**TIPS AND TRICKS**

- Don't sag your belly; lift your belly button to the sky to give your lower back support.
- Don't forget to firm up your fanny; put a thousand dollar bill between your butt cheeks —well, at least imagine it!

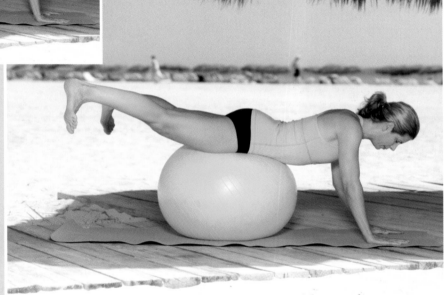

**POSITION 1:** Inhale to open your legs as wide as you can. Exhale to close your legs, engaging your inner thighs and booty. If you need a rest, drape yourself over the ball after you're done and just breathe. It's a yummy lower back stretch.

## THE PAYOFF:

Tightens your tushie and inner thighs.

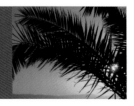

# Froggy with Big Ball

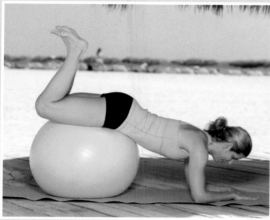

**STARTING POSITION:** Roll onto your hips so the ball supports your torso. Place your elbows on the floor in front of the ball and then open your legs slightly to bend your knees, placing your heels together. Gaze at the floor.

### TIPS AND TRICKS

- Don't sag your belly; lift your belly button to the sky to give your lower back support.

- Don't forget to firm up your fanny; put a thousand dollar bill between your butt cheeks —well, at least imagine it!

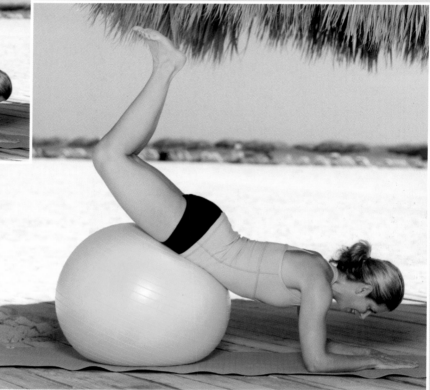

**POSITION 1:** Inhale to lift your feet to the ceiling, and then exhale to lower your knees to the ball. If you need a rest, drape yourself over the ball after you're done and just breathe. It's a yummy lower back stretch.

## THE PAYOFF:

Makes for a serious booty buster.

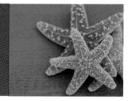

# Inner Thigh Squeeze with Big Ball

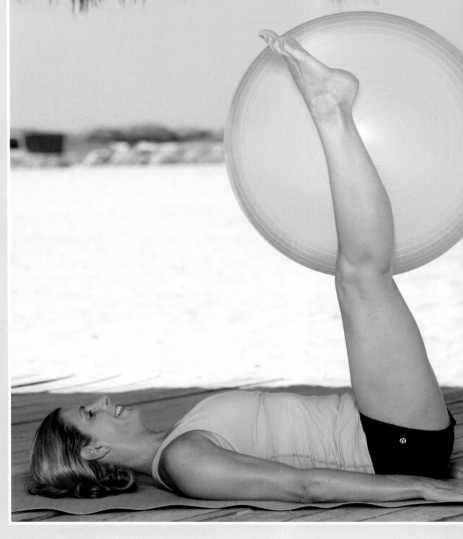

**STARTING POSITION:** Lie on your back with your legs at a 90-degree angle and straighten your arms by your sides. Place the ball between your thighs; squeeze and release; squeeze and release.

**TIPS AND TRICKS**

- Don't droop your foot; make sure your toes are in line with your knees and your knees are in line with your hips.

- Don't forget to squeeze from your knees only; squeeze like mad so you get the delicious inner thigh work!

## THE PAYOFF:

Gives you gorgeous inner thighs.

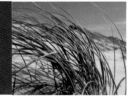

## THURSDAY: BECOMING FABULOUS WITH BOOT-CAMP-STRENGTH INTERVALS

Today, repeat Monday's boot camp workout, p. 253.

## FRIDAY: GETTING BIKINI LEAN WITH STEADY-STATE CARDIO

Today, repeat Tuesday's cardio workout, p. 266.

## SATURDAY: BUSTING YOUR BOOTY WITH PILATES

Today, repeat Wednesday's Pilates workout, p. 266.

## SUNDAY: CELEBRATE YOU!

Well, you're done! I hope you feel amazing and have the confidence to show off those curves. Life is too short not to wear a bikini and celebrate your body. Keep going—you can repeat any of these workouts and expect even more amazing results—leaner legs and a tighter tush. Have fun in the sun!

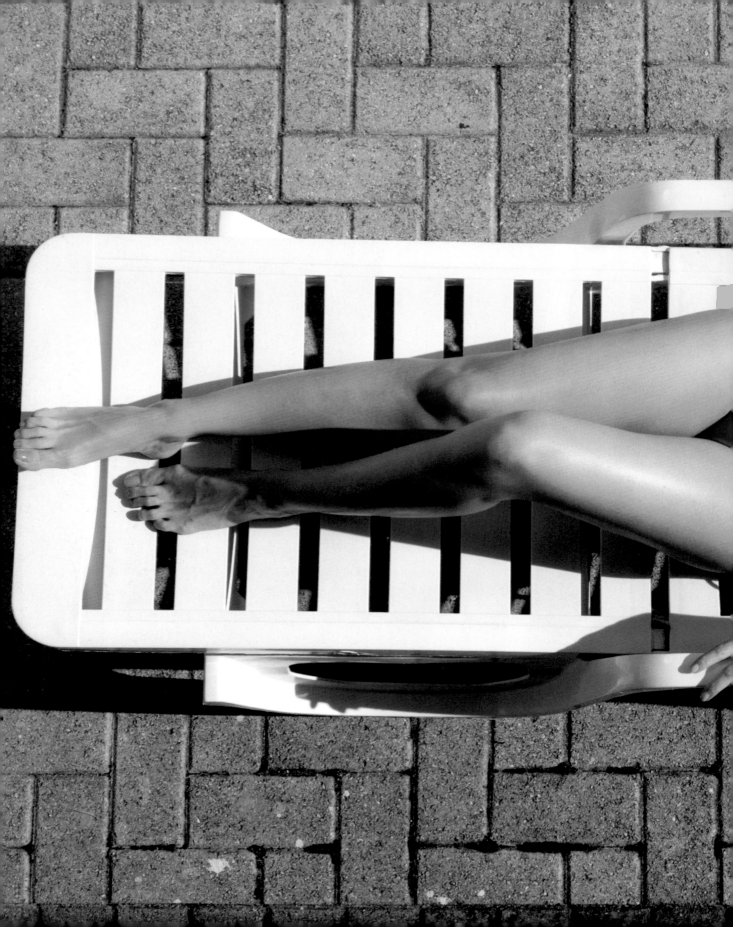

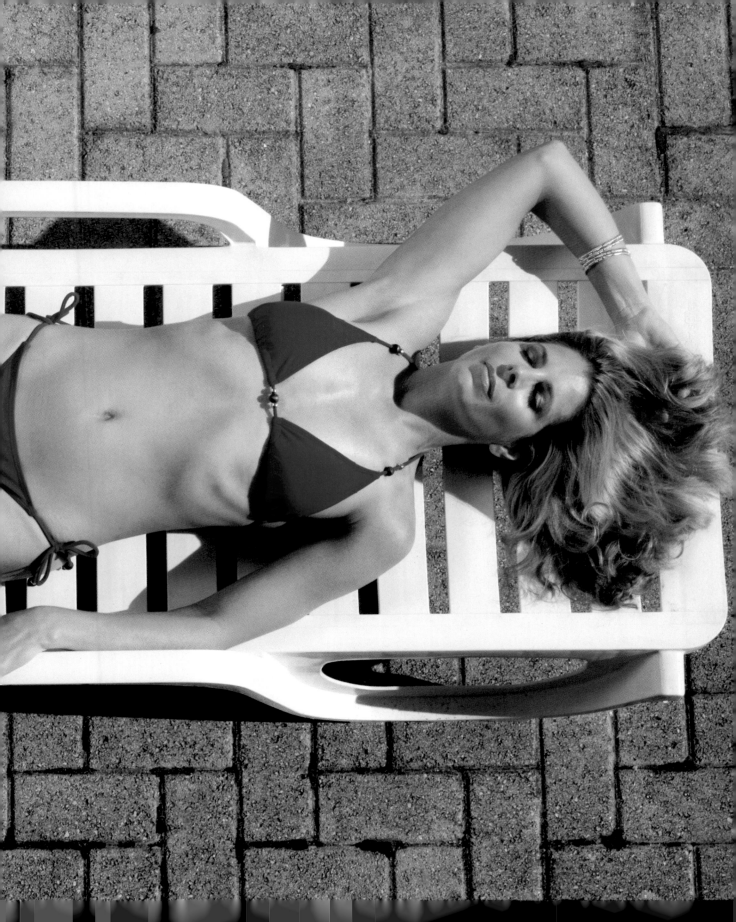

# List of Exercises

# List of Exercises

# List of Exercises

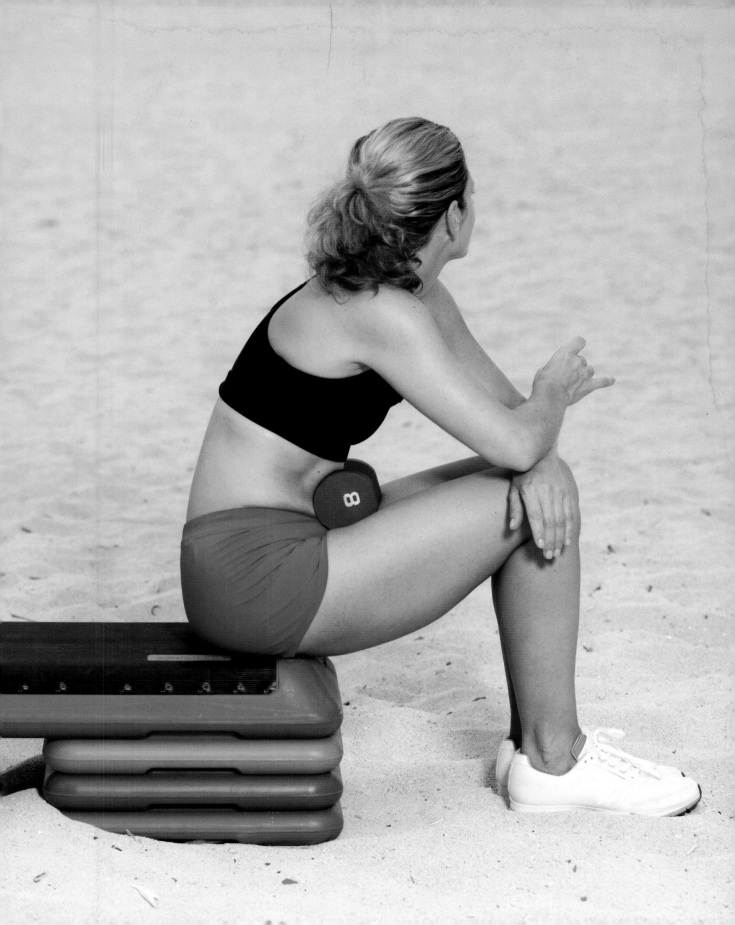

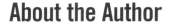

## About the Author

You can watch Karon Karter teach Pilates in her new Pilates television series, *Pilates from the Inside Out*. She also has eight health and fitness books under her belt. Her most recent publication, *Balance Training: Stability Workouts for Core Strength and a Sculpted Body*, is Amazon's top pick for new books. Her book *Pilates Lite* is now sold in five languages. Her other publications include *The Complete Idiot's Guide to Body Ball Illustrated*, *The Core Strength Workout*, *The Complete Idiot's Guide to Pilates*, *The Complete Idiot's Guide to Kickboxing*, and *The Healthy Flier: How to Protect Yourself From the Hidden Hazards of Airline Travel*.

Ms. Karter has also been featured in major newspapers nationwide, including *The New York Times*, *The Miami Herald*, *The Seattle Times*, and *The Dallas Morning News*. Her books have been publicized in national magazines such as *The National Enquirer*, *The Bottom Line*, *PilatesStyle*, *Modern Bride*, *Health*, and *Self*. In addition, she has made several appearances on local morning news shows such as *Good Morning Texas*, *Good Day Texas*, and *Fox News*.

Ms. Karter was *Self* magazine's core strength expert for their Self Challenge 2004, in which her book, *The Core Strength Workout*, was featured. She was guest author on Visions Women's Expo, and Barnes and Noble featured her books and selected her as the "Author of the Month" in January 2005. Ms. Karter has fifteen years of experience in the fitness and health industry and she interned and then worked for Dr. Kenneth Cooper's Institute for Aerobic Research, where she supervised new corporate health programs, including Dow Chemical's "Up with Life" and Texas Instruments' "Life Track." Her certifications include Physical Fitness Specialist and Group Leadership Training from the Aerobics Institute; Resist-a-Ball training; Ashtanga (yoga) training with Manju Jois; Pilates certification from the classically trained Glenn Studio; and Beryl Bender Birch Ashtanga certification. Currently, she teaches Pilates and has influenced the fitness lives of thousands of students.